LABORS OF LOVE

Labors of Love

Nursing Homes and the Structures of Care Work

Jason Rodriquez

NEW YORK UNIVERSITY PRESS
New York and London

NEW YORK UNIVERSITY PRESS
New York and London
www.nyupress.org

References to Internet websites (URLs) were accurate at the time of writing.
Neither the author nor New York University Press is responsible for URLs that
may have expired or changed since the manuscript was prepared.

LIBRARY OF CONGRESS CATALOGING-IN-PUBLICATION DATA
Rodriquez, Jason, 1978- author.
Labors of love : nursing homes and the structures of care work / Jason Rodriquez.
p. ; cm.
Includes bibliographical references and index.
ISBN 978-1-4798-3940-7 (cloth : alk. paper) -- ISBN 978-1-4798-6430-0 (paper : alk. paper)
I. Title.
[DNLM: 1. Aged--United States. 2. Nursing Homes--organization & administration--
United States. 3. Geriatric Nursing--methods--United States. 4. Health Services for the
Aged--organization & administration--United States. 5. Nursing Homes--manpower--
United States. 6. Reimbursement Mechanisms--organization & administration--United
States. WT 27 AA1]
RA997
362.16--dc23
2014018128

New York University Press books are printed on acid-free paper,
and their binding materials are chosen for strength and durability.
We strive to use environmentally responsible suppliers and materials
to the greatest extent possible in publishing our books.

Manufactured in the United States of America

10 9 8 7 6 5 4 3 2 1

Also available as an ebook

This book is dedicated to my grandmother,

Mary T. Rodriquez

CONTENTS

ACKNOWLEDGMENTS

Writing is both an analytic and a collaborative process. Many friends, colleagues, advisors, and audiences contributed ideas and gave advice that
helped me write this book, and I would like to acknowledge how grateful I
am for their support. At the University of Massachusetts–Amherst, I became
a sociologist under the guidance of Robert Zussman. I am deeply indebted
to him for many reasons, not least among them that he taught me how to
start and then finish a project. Bob's enormously creative insights continue to
inspire me. Naomi Gerstel helped me figure out what this project was about,
offering exceptionally helpful advice in its early stages. I am thankful for her
unwavering support and for sticking with me when I was (am) difficult. Dan
Clawson taught me the mechanics of doing research, and I am fortunate to
have had the opportunity to work with him. Don Tomaskovic-Devey and
Joya Misra are tremendous role models whom I admire greatly. I appreciate
all of their supportive advice and encouragement. I also appreciate the assistance of Cynthia Jacelon, whose perspective as a scholar-nurse added a lot
to my thinking about the issues. Early on at UMass I benefitted from working with Jill McCorkel and Gianpaolo Baiocchi; even though their research
addresses totally different issues than those I am concerned with in this book,
I was inspired by their sociological imaginations and learned a lot from them.
Karen Mason provided important logistical support as I collected the data.

As an NIMH Postdoctoral Fellow at the Institute for Health, Health
Care Policy, and Aging Research at Rutgers University, I had the opportunity to think about my research in new ways. The institute provided valuable resources and time as I revised and refined this book. I would especially
like to thank Deborah Carr, Allan Horwitz, and David Mechanic. Their
insightful comments on chapter drafts and timely career advice have been
immensely helpful. I learned a lot from my colleagues at the institute and am
happy to have shared the experience with Joanne Hash, Azure Thompson,
and R. Tyson Smith. The Sociology Department at the University of Missouri–Columbia has been a great place to finish this book. Special thanks
to Wayne Brekhus, Jaber Gubrium, Joan Hermsen, Erica Morales, and Amit

Prasad. I also wish to thank Margaret Ralston, Mike Sickels, and the graduate students in my spring 2012 seminar on Qualitative Methodology for pushing me to think harder about how the methodological choices I made shaped what I could say in this book, and how I could say it.

The staff of the two nursing homes researched for this book graciously allowed me access into their worlds. I am eternally grateful for their openness and trust in me to accurately represent their experiences. I would also like to thank the National Science Foundation and the Research Council at the University of Missouri–Columbia for their generous financial support of this project. Thank you to Ilene Kalish and the entire staff at New York University Press. Ilene believed in the book from our very first meeting, and that helped me believe in it too. Joseph Dahm did an excellent job with the final copyedit.

Throughout the long process of writing this book, I received valuable comments and advice from many other people. I would especially like to thank Harvey Bergholz, Rob Brandt, Gary Alan Fine, Suzanne Gordon, Steven Lopez, Arnold Relman, Mark Schlesinger, and Frank Thompson. I have great friends who are also professional colleagues, and this book is better because of the immensely enjoyable conversations with them about this project and many other sociological matters. I cherish my friendships with Brittnie Aiello, Dustin Avent-Holt, Sarah Becker, Josh Carreiro, Mark Gammon, Ben Johnson, Rachel Rybaczuk, Kelan Steel-Lowney, and Amy Wilkins. Finally, I want to thank my wife, Kim Johnson, who was with me every step of the way. She has been endlessly supportive, from the very beginning when this book was little more than a vague idea all the way through to writing its final passages. In the moments when I thought I would never finish it, or that nobody would read it, her boundless enthusiasm gave me the motivation to keep going and the confidence to believe that this book has been worth the time and effort.

Introduction

Locating Nursing Home Care Work

"Jason is helping me out, so he can hear all of this," said Andy Fischer, the administrator of Rolling Hills Extended Care and Rehabilitation Center, a nonprofit and secular nursing home. Eli, a sick old man with shaggy white hair and thick glasses, pedaled his wheelchair until he came to a standstill in Andy's doorway. Eli looked tired and somewhat disheveled, wearing an over-sized red-and-black flannel shirt, gray cotton shorts, white socks pulled up toward his knees, and an old pair of loafers. His right arm was held in a sling that looked uncomfortable. Andy leaned forward in his office chair, elbows on his knees, and explained to Eli that his check for "room and board" had bounced for the fourth consecutive month. In his typically informal and homespun style, Andy asked Eli, "What's going on dude?"

Eli was not sure. He knew he was "behind on the rent," but did not know why; his daughter was supposed to pay the nursing home with his pension checks. She assumed control over his finances after he moved into Rolling Hills about a year earlier. Later, Andy wondered aloud to me whether Eli's daughter took his money for herself, which he claimed happened more than occasionally. But during the meeting, Eli told Andy that his daughter had a doctorate in chemistry and "could buy you and me," defending his daughter against the implication that she was pocketing his money. Andy too did not understand how Eli had been allowed to fall so far behind, and commented, "It's clear you two aren't on the same page." Andy suggested that Eli make Rolling Hills his representative payee, which meant that the nursing home would receive his pension and Social Security checks directly, pay his "room and board," then deposit what remained into a personal funds account. Eli agreed, or perhaps he acquiesced. Then, upon leaving, he turned to wheel out of Andy's doorway and noticed his friend and co-resident nearby. He explained sarcastically, "I just got called to the principal's office." Andy closed the door. I told him that I felt bad for Eli. Andy squinted in disbelief and shook his head. "No," he huffed, "you should feel bad for me. He hasn't paid us in four months!" Yet a few minutes later, when Andy had cooled down a bit, he confided to me that he never wanted to pursue money from residents.

In fact, he explained that this was why he left the for-profit nursing home side of the industry for the nonprofit sector. Now, just a few years later, he found himself in the unenviable position of carrying out the same business practices he fled from, except this time it was as the administrator of a non-profit nursing home.

I met Andy for the first time on a chilly, sunny November afternoon in New England. Expecting my arrival, he greeted me warmly just inside the foyer of Rolling Hills, a two-story brick building with white columns that provided nursing home services for about 120 individuals, a bit more than the national average. He was tall, with reddish-blonde hair styled high to make him appear even taller. His size was matched by his demonstrative personality: outgoing, affable, and spontaneous. Initially, I sent him a letter to introduce myself and to outline my project. I followed up with a phone call a few days later. Looking back and considering how infrequently he sat at his desk, I am grateful and lucky he was there to answer the phone. I told him of my interest in understanding the role of emotions in nursing home care work. Throughout the eighteen months I spent conducting field research at Rolling Hills, and at the other nursing home researched for this book, Golden Bay, I continued to pursue the issue of emotions in nursing homes, but Andy led me to thinking about emotions within the context of the financial and regulatory structures that shape nursing home care work.

Andy told me that his time as the administrator at for-profit nursing homes led him to conclude that their day-to-day decision making was overly oriented toward cost-efficiency at the expense of resident quality of life. In fact, he was called to account for expenses that were over budget by as little as a few hundred dollars. Andy's supervisor at his last for-profit facility, an investor-owned and nationally recognized for-profit corporation, was, in his words, "focused like a laser on the bottom line." Andy was stunned when his supervisor required that he develop a plan to discharge a half-dozen Medicaid residents. Andy was told to replace them with individuals whose care would be more financially lucrative for the facility. Medicaid pays the lowest, less than individuals who pay for care from their savings and much less than people whose care is paid by Medicare. Medicare, although not designed to reimburse for nursing home care, will pay "skilled nursing facilities" such as nursing homes for up to one hundred days of physical, occupational, or speech rehabilitation, and at much higher rates than any other form of payment. The Medicaid residents were poor, or more likely became poor paying for nursing home care out of pocket. The nursing home was truly their *home*, and Andy did not want to discharge them. This, he claimed, was the moment he decided to leave behind the for-profit nursing home sector and seek out work at a nonprofit.

The small nonprofit company that owned Rolling Hills, he said, would never force him to discharge Medicaid residents, whose care generates much lower reimbursements than that of Medicare residents and residents who pay privately from their life savings. He regarded nursing home administration at Rolling Hills as an altogether different enterprise than what he had done at the for-profits. For one thing, he had greater discretion to make decisions based on what was best for the residents' care. When he became the administrator at Rolling Hills, he replaced all the mattresses because they were outdated and potentially hazardous. The mattresses had springs inside that posed an unacceptably high risk of pressure ulcers, also known as "bedsores," which are lesions caused by prolonged periods of unrelieved pressure on the body. Although they are preventable and treatable if caught early, they can quickly progress and become fatal, particularly among the elderly. State and federal regulators use the number of pressure ulcers acquired by residents as a key metric of nursing home quality. Replacing the mattresses was an expensive upgrade, which he pointed to as evidence that the facility was oriented toward good care, even though it cost a lot of money. In addition to the new mattresses, he bought new equipment, organized trainings, prioritized outreach to potential volunteer networks and local media, and worked to improve the organizational culture with a rhetoric of "teamwork," the idea that everyone works together toward the common goal of quality care. He set the tone to his staff that the facility would do something different from—and for that matter better than—the for-profits that dominated the local market.

Rolling Hills engaged, initially, in various forms of altruistic and community-oriented activities, while Golden Bay Nursing and Rehabilitation Center, the other nursing home I researched for this book, operated from a corporate model premised on profitability and cost-efficiency. Golden Bay was part of an investor-owned, nationwide, for-profit chain that operated hundreds of health services organizations across the country. It aggressively expanded and purchased subsidiaries to vertically integrate rehabilitation therapy services and medical staffing agencies. Cynthia Rosen had been the administrator there for several years and was highly regarded by her immediate staff because she provided stable and consistent leadership. She was proud of the facility and boasted not only that it was profitable, but that it had become increasingly so in the years under her management. Cynthia had a calm, warm presence. She was friendly but spoke carefully and seemed to keep in the back of her mind that anything she said around me could be published. Smart and conscientious, she was recognized as a top administrator in the company perhaps because she closely monitored the financial indicators of the nursing home, especially the "case mix," meaning the proportions of residents whose care was reimbursed by Medicare or paid privately out of pocket to balance against Medicaid residents. Medicaid reimburses nursing homes for care at rates that are often lower than the operational costs to house these individuals.

In my first meeting with Andy, I was convinced. The story he told was one I was ready to hear, a story about the superiority of nonprofits to proprietary nursing homes, of altruism and compassion to crass profit seeking. I still think this today, but, having spent considerable time in nursing homes, I now also realize that the story is much more complicated than Andy described. This book is about how Andy and Cynthia managed their nursing homes given the financial and regulatory demands of the nursing home industry, but it is about much more than that. It is about the complex minuet nursing home staff dance between a logic of care and a logic of cost. The structure of the nursing home industry imposes on care workers, constraining them into a range of behavior and thought patterns that objectify residents as embodiments of reimbursable activities. Given these unwanted constraints, staff turned to the emotional rewards of care work to make the labor bearable. Many of them told me they continued to work in nursing homes because they loved the residents and loved caring for people who needed them. The harsh structural constraints of these workplaces, providing low pay and minimal prestige, unenforced workplace protections, and almost no opportunities for meaningful career advancement, were enough to make many nursing home care workers move on for other work. Those who stayed were a kind of "prisoner of love," as Paula England put it.[1] Their love for residents was the main reason they continued to do nursing home care work, despite the otherwise unrewarding work environment.

Workers in the Nursing Home Industry

Nursing homes are typically composed of rigid vertical hierarchies in which floor staff do the direct face-to-face care work with residents and are paid on an hourly basis while salaried managers attend primarily to financial and regulatory matters. Part of the appeal of studying care work in nursing homes is that, with an average size of about one hundred beds, they are small enough to gain the perspectives of employees throughout the workplace yet large enough also to gain insights into how the rigid lines of authority and supervision structure the experience. The majority of workers in the "service theater," to use Rachel Sherman's phrase,[2] are certified nursing assistants.

Of the 16 million workers in the health care sector, more than 1.5 million of them are certified nursing assistants, and this number is expected to grow by 20 percent between 2010 and 2020, making nursing assistants among the top twenty fastest growing occupations in the United States. Almost half of nursing assistants work in nursing homes, while the rest typically work in hospitals, clinics, or doctors' offices. Many also work as home health aides. Nursing assistant is an entry-level position in health care that requires little training. In the state where this research was conducted, trainees were required to take a one-hundred-hour course and then pass a certification exam before they were allowed to work as a certified nursing assistant. Beyond that, nursing assistants face dim prospects for career advancement, and most tend to move laterally across nursing homes rather than vertically up the chain of command. The median wage for nursing assistants, according to the Bureau of Labor Statistics,[3] is eleven dollars per hour (twenty-four thousand dollars annually), and moreover, they face unstable work schedules and difficult working conditions. They are at elevated risk for workplace injuries because they lift and turn residents frequently, making them particularly susceptible to lower back and wrist injuries. They are also exposed to infections, diseases, and physically, verbally, and sexually aggressive behavior from agitated residents.[4] These are some of the reasons why the turnover rate among nursing assistants in nursing homes is extremely high.[5]

There have been a handful of exemplary ethnographies of nursing homes that have given voice to nursing assistants and sought to highlight the ways that they manage the strains of their work within the bureaucratic and hierarchical structure of nursing homes.[6] As important as these studies have been, they have had the tendency to overlook all the other nursing home care workers. These individuals include dietary aides, activities assistants, rehabilitation aides, social workers, and maintenance staff. Less is known about these workers, but all of them are important to a functioning nursing home. This book integrates their experiences to provide a fuller portrait of nursing homes as workplaces.

The demographic characteristics of the floor staff in this study are largely consistent with the national picture of nursing home care workers. In 2004 the Centers for Disease Control and Prevention conducted their first nationally representative survey of certified nursing assistants who work in nursing homes as part of their National Nursing Home Survey. The survey found that 92 percent of nursing assistants are women, more than 80 percent are over the age of twenty-five, and almost 75 percent have a high school diploma or less education. Nationally, nursing assistants working in nursing homes are disproportionally black, representing 38 percent of all these workers. About

53 percent of nursing assistants are white. Due to the location of these nursing homes, almost all of the staff members and residents at Rolling Hills and Golden Bay were white. At the level of nursing assistants, Golden Bay had a bit more racial and ethnic diversity than Rolling Hills. A handful of Latinas worked at Golden Bay as nursing assistants. Golden Bay was located close enough to a town that had a large Latino/a population, while Rolling Hills was farther away and in a somewhat more rural area. Golden Bay recruited nursing assistants from the town, while Rolling Hills tended to hire staff from the white farming communities that surrounded the area. The differences in ethnic composition that existed between the two facilities did not extend above the nursing assistant level on the work hierarchy. In other words, Golden Bay had a handful of Latina nursing assistants, but nearly all others at both nursing homes were white women.

The nursing department primarily comprises nursing assistants, but licensed practical nurses (LPNs) and registered nurses (RNs) also work on the nursing home floor. LPNs have less nursing education than RNs, but in nursing homes they often do the same work: they dispense medication to residents and monitor the nursing assistants. LPNs and RNs make up 13 percent and 8 percent, respectively, of the nursing home workforce. In total, 28 percent of LPNs and only 5 percent of nurses work in nursing homes; many nurses are likely lured away from nursing home care for jobs in hospitals that pay more and often entail more autonomy and better benefits. Like nursing assistants, LPN and RN occupations are expected to grow rapidly, between 20 and 25 percent over the next ten years according to the Bureau of Labor Statistics.[7] The median annual salary of an LPN working in a nursing home is forty thousand dollars, much more than nursing assistants' salaries but much less compared to RNs in nursing homes, who earn a median salary of fifty-seven thousand dollars. This is likely due to the fact that LPNs have fewer opportunities for career advancement compared to RNs. An RN must sign most state forms, limiting the possibility that LPNs will become managers.

Managers at Rolling Hills and Golden Bay were mostly women nurses, but the maintenance directors at both nursing homes were men. Andy, the administrator at Rolling Hills, was an outlier in a few respects, in that he was neither a woman nor a nurse. He started his career as a volunteer and eventually took college courses in health services that were designed to train students to become nursing home administrators. Andy's supervisor also was a man, and both companies were run by men, so it is possible if not likely that Andy benefited from a "glass escalator" effect, whereby men quickly ascend organizational hierarchies in fields that are traditionally associated with women's work.[8]

Health care is one of the fastest growing industries in the U.S. economy, and the Bureau of Labor Statistics projects that ten of the twenty fastest growing occupations over the next decade will be in the health care industry.[9] As the baby boomer generation enters retirement and life expectancy lengthens, the number of workers needed to provide long-term care will increase sharply. The number of people over the age of sixty-five is projected to double by 2030, but in terms of nursing home care, the larger issue may be that the number of individuals over the age of eighty-five, currently about five million, is expected to surge to twenty million by 2050.[10] Individuals over age eighty-five are the most likely to require continuous care in institutional settings and currently make up more than half of the nursing home population. The demand for nursing assistants, home health care aids, physical and occupational therapists, and others who will provide care to the elderly will grow dramatically in the coming decades. These jobs cannot be outsourced to workers overseas.

Just as most studies of nursing home care work focus on the experience of nursing assistants at the bottom of the work hierarchy, studies that discuss management tend to focus narrowly on administrators and nursing directors. This book is more inclusive, incorporating the perspectives of reimbursement coordinators, financial managers, unit staff managers, and various other supervisors who are central organizational actors in nursing homes. Managers were typically RNs who had "paid their dues" working shifts on the nursing home floor before moving up to a salaried position with an office, removed from the daily grind of direct care work for a position centrally focused on reimbursement and regulatory matters.

The Research

The data gathered for this book are the result of eighteen months of fieldwork at two nursing homes and sixty-five interviews with their staff members. I gained access to Rolling Hills Extended Care and Rehabilitation in November 2006. Located on a hilly side street near a highway, it was separated from the street by about a hundred yards of grass and light forest. The facility was housed in a several-decades-old brick building shaped like a T. Just inside was a big, octagonal foyer leading to the front hallway. The carpeted, wallpapered halls were often decorated to reflect an upcoming holiday, especially in December, when the staff invited residents and their families to decorate the large plastic Christmas tree and place Hanukkah decorations. There were small couches and chairs that friends and family used to chat with their loved ones away from the noise and energy on the units. The company newsletter and a calendar with upcoming events sat atop a small, round wooden table in the center of the room. In the corner, on a smaller wooden table, lay the results from the most recent inspection by the Department of Public Health, which by law must be easily accessible to the public. After passing through the entryway, managers' offices lined the front hallway that led to the facility's main thoroughfare. The dining room, activities office, and rehabilitation gym were located off this central artery that connected the units. The locked doors to the dementia unit were at one end, while the subacute rehabilitation unit was at the other end. The residents on the long-term care unit lived upstairs. The floors throughout the facility were carpeted with a pattern designed to hide stains, and the walls were either painted or wallpapered and had large wooden handrails to assist residents in case they lost their balance. The hallways were spacious and easily fit two wheelchairs across. The doors to residents' rooms often remained open throughout the day, as residents were lined up, sitting in their wheelchairs, gathered around the nursing stations in the middle of the units.

A few months after I started collecting data at the nonprofit Rolling Hills, Andy helped me gain access to Golden Bay Nursing and Rehabilitation Center, which was part of a large, national for-profit chain of health care facilities. He knew Cynthia, the administrator, through professional networks and called her on my behalf. Several days later I spoke to her by phone and we set up a meeting. When we met, she kindly agreed to allow me one month of participant observation and then she would determine how much more time, if any, I could spend at the facility. We never had that meeting. She later explained that she let me stay because I did not interfere with the work being done in the nursing home.

Golden Bay was built around the same time as Rolling Hills and had a very similar look and layout. Its parking lot and brick building were set away from the road by about a hundred yards of grass and a handful of maple trees. A receptionist monitored the large white doors and greeted all visitors, who had to sign in before they were permitted to proceed. The small foyer of the facility had a gently worn love seat, a few stately chairs, and a large vase filled with fake flowers sitting atop a table. A rarely played baby grand piano sat along the wall. After signing in with the receptionist, visitors walked through another large white door to the front hallway, which, like at Rolling Hills, was where most of the managers' offices were located. Golden Bay looked very similar to Rolling Hills on the outside but inside seemed a bit more worn and darker. Doors to both residents' rooms and staff offices were more likely to be closed at Golden Bay than at Rolling Hills. About a month after I arrived at Golden Bay, I was offered a small desk and chair in the facility's reimbursement office, which I accepted, and it served as something of a home base.

On most days at Golden Bay, a long table with candy and baked goods for sale stood in the middle of the central hallway. Two residents spent their day "working" at the tabletop store and chatting with people. The building's layout was essentially the same as Rolling Hills', except for the rehabilitation gym. It was roughly twice the size of the one at Rolling Hills. It also had more modern equipment and staff. This allowed Golden Bay to generate more revenue from Medicare, which reimburses nursing homes for up to one hundred days of rehabilitative care (after a three-night qualifying hospital stay) at rates that often exceed five hundred dollars per day, much more than Medicaid reimbursements, which are typically under two hundred dollars per day for as long as the individual resides. In addition to the rehabilitation gym, the activities room, the dining room, a hairdresser, a small store run by activities assistants, and a small library were connected to Golden Bay's central hallway.

Both nursing homes had three nursing units: a subacute rehabilitation unit for individuals who had been discharged recently from a hospital and were at the nursing home to gain strength and recover abilities that would allow them to go home, a long-term care unit for people who could no longer live independently safely, and a locked unit for people with severe dementia. The rehabilitation unit had by far the fastest pace and had the highest resident turnover, as individuals often started in a wheelchair, then regained enough strength to walk with the assistance of a cane or walker, and then finally regained enough abilities to leave the nursing home and return to their place of residence. This unit had quite a bit of foot traffic; family members, physicians, psychiatrists, and physical, occupational, and speech therapists were there every day. This unit was also the most important financially, as the high-reimbursement Medicare residents were housed there. It stood in striking contrast to the dementia unit, which had the slowest pace and the most stable daily routine. It had very few visitors and felt self-contained compared to the others. Almost all of the individuals living on this unit were on Medicaid, typically after "spending down" their accumulated life savings paying for the nursing home out of pocket. On the long-term care unit, residents had stable daily routines, but the pace on the unit was more active than that on the dementia unit and there were more visitors. Residents on the long-term care unit may have had some symptoms of dementia but required assistance with daily activities that they could not easily do themselves.

My fieldwork allowed me to gain access to the character and contours of work from many angles. I conducted participant observation between two and four days a week, usually in four-hour stretches. Typically, I arrived in the morning before the daily managers meeting and left sometime in the afternoon after lunch. After a few months I began to observe evening shifts to get a sense of temporal variation, but I usually visited during the day so I could attend meetings. In the summer of 2007 I increased the extent of my fieldwork and began to conduct interviews with staff. In the fall of 2007, I scaled my observations back to presummer levels and conducted interviews up until fieldwork concluded in the spring of 2008. I spent time observing in and around nursing stations and shadowing nursing assistants and licensed nursing staff, and I occasionally lent a hand with serving meals or escorting residents to activities, to the rehabilitation gym, and to meals in the main hall. I helped out informally as a volunteer activities assistant. I often spent several consecutive hours on the units to get a good sense of the pace of the daily routine. To hear informal conversation between staff, I observed in break rooms and at holiday parties and other staff functions, and I spent time having lunch or loitering outside at the "butt hut" with staff on smoking breaks. I routinely observed staff meetings, including the daily managers meetings, nursing reports, care plan meetings, Medicare meetings, employee retention committee meetings, and staff trainings. In addition, I had innumerable conversations with various individuals in the organizations, from the maintenance staff to the activities aides, physical, occupational, and speech therapy staff, dietary aides, residents, and visitors. I recorded my observations in detailed field notes written soon after I left the facility. To recall events accurately, I jotted down quotes or keywords in unobtrusive spots and expanded on them at the end of each day.

Approximately six months after I began fieldwork at Rolling Hills I conducted the first of sixty-five staff interviews. I asked everyone I interviewed a core set of questions, although the interviews varied according to my observations and were tailored to each individual, occupation, and organization. I interviewed staff members throughout the organizational chain, including certified nursing assistants, LPNs, RNs, physical therapists, occupational therapists, speech therapists, social workers, activities assistants, unit managers, directors of nursing, and the administrators. Please see Table I.1 for a list of key staff members who appear in the book and Figure I.1 for a flow chart of the organizational structure of the nursing homes. Conducting interviews in the middle stage of my fieldwork allowed for time to build rapport with staff members and to gain knowledge of particular events that I wanted to learn more about. I asked staff members about their daily job tasks, their work history, the emotional attachments they had with residents (or not), how the documentation and

Table I.1. Key Staff Members

Rolling Hills (Nonprofit)		Golden Bay (For-Profit)	
Staff	Job Title	Staff	Job Title
Managers		Managers	
Mike	Regional Administrator	Cynthia	Administrator
Andy	Administrator	Lucy	Director of Nursing
Joanne	Director of Nursing	Crystal	Medicaid Reimbursement Coordinator
Nancy	Staff Development Coordinator	Patricia	Staff Development Coordinator
Victoria	Medicaid Reimbursement Coordinator	Francine	Admissions Coordinator
Beverly	Admissions Coordinator	Barbara	Clinical Case Coordinator
Flo	Dietary Manager	Heather	Long-Term Care Unit Manager
Dawn	Subacute Rehabilitation Unit Manager	Ruby	Financial Manager
Carol	Medicare Reimbursement Coordinator	Debby	Dementia Unit Manager
Jamie	Social Services Director	Kirsten	Rehabilitation Coordinator
Liz	Activities Manager	Susan	Social Services Director
Tina	Scheduler	Dorothea	Care Plan Coordinator
		Dave	Maintenance Director
		Terry	Activities Manager
Floor Staff		Floor Staff	
Stephanie	Nurse	Carla	Nurse
Caryn	Nurse	Carissa	Nurse
Cindy	Nursing Assistant	Megan	Nurse
Maria	Nursing Assistant	Louise	Nurse
Bonnie	Nursing Assistant	Ariel	Nurse
Daphne	Nursing Assistant	Stacey	Nurse/Wound Care Manager
Caroline	Nursing Assistant	Doris	Nursing Assistant
Angela	Nursing Assistant	Laura	Nursing Assistant
Alice	Nursing Assistant	Frankie	Nursing Assistant
Diane	Nursing Assistant		
Rebecca	Nursing Assistant		
Jamie	Nursing Assistant		
Randi	Activities Assistant		
Marlene	Activities Assistant		
Dotty	Activities Assistant		

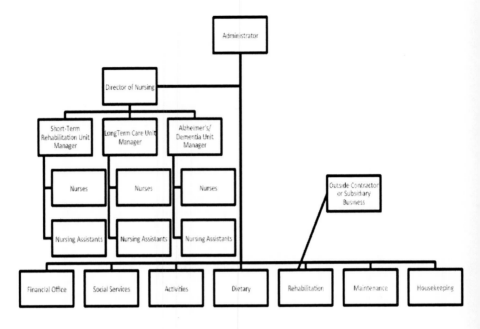

Figure I.1. Flow Chart of Organizational Structure of the Nursing Homes

reimbursement process shaped their work, the problems and challenges they faced on the job, and what it felt like to care for people who often died in their care. The individuals I interviewed ranged in age from their early twenties to their mid-seventies, and given the substantial differences in pay between floor staff and managers, there was a fair degree of class variation. Other staff demographics were fairly consistent with the makeup of the residents. Most residents were white elderly women, whereas the floor staff at Rolling Hills tended to be white women in their thirties or forties and at Golden Bay mostly white women, with some Latinas, in their twenties or thirties.

In addition to the observations and staff interviews, I collected financial records, brochures, advertisements, various internal documents, and other forms of material culture produced by both nursing homes. These documents are useful inasmuch as they reveal the kind of image the facilities tried to propagate about themselves. They were key parts of the narratives that each facility crafted about what they believed about themselves and what they aspired to be. I also utilized data collected by state and federal regulatory agencies. These agencies, primarily the Centers for Medicare and

Medicaid Services (CMS) and the state Department of Public Health, routinely collect data on the characteristics of nursing home populations and the performance of the facilities. I used these data to check or clarify claims made by the nursing home managers and, where I could, examine how far and wide the findings of this study generalize to nursing homes across the country. Combining these sources of data—field observations, documents, and interviews—allowed me to triangulate sources and strengthen the evidentiary base of the research.[11]

I utilized multiple layers of camouflage to protect the confidentiality of the participants in this study. I have changed the names of all study participants and the organizations. I also am vague about certain details that could have provided even more context and detail but would have opened the possibility that the individuals or the nursing homes could be identified. Last, I have altered certain details about people and the nursing homes that are not critical to the arguments but do provide context, such as the physical appearance of the participants and of the nursing homes.

Nursing Home Care Work

Medicaid and Medicare pay nursing homes on a fee-for-service basis, meaning the more services they provide and bill for, the more reimbursement money they receive. The Patient Protection and Affordable Care Act makes some changes to the reimbursement system that will encourage health services organizations to increase the value instead of the volume of services provided. For example, CMS now imposes financial penalties on the 25 percent of hospitals that have the highest rates of hospital-acquired conditions such as infections and bedsores. But those changes apply much more to hospitals than they do to nursing homes. What remains is a nursing home industry, like the larger health care system it is a piece of, that is deeply driven by profit and incentivized to provide more care, even though more care is not necessarily better care.[12] The profitability of nursing home care relies, to a great extent, on doing a lot of work on residents. The fee-for-service model of reimbursement to nursing homes means that nursing homes get reimbursed more when residents are more dependent on staff for everyday activities like getting dressed and eating. This lucrative payment model has helped to generate a system in which presently more than two-thirds of the nation's sixteen thousand nursing homes operate as for-profit facilities and more than half are part of a multifacility chain. About one-quarter are nonprofit, and the rest are publicly owned and operated.[13] Private equity groups have noticed the opportunities for quick profits, buying up nursing homes, often with complex management structures that obscure ultimate responsibility for residents' care and safety.[14]

Yet the big story about health care over the past couple of decades has not been so much about the rise of the for-profit sector (although that is certainly an important story) but more about nonprofits coming to act like for-profits—about the successful imposition of a "market regime" on a sector of the economy that had previously been shielded from such pressures. As Paul Starr wrote in his landmark study *The Social Transformation of American Medicine*, "The organizational culture of medicine used to be dominated by the ideals of professionalism and voluntarism, which softened the underlying acquisitive activity."[15] But that is no longer the case. Medical payment and regulatory systems are, self-consciously, policy instruments meant to encourage some activities and discourage others. There is plenty of evidence that reimbursement incentives do shape the behavior of health services organizations, but with very little sense of the processes by which these broad policy contexts are expressed in everyday practices. The stories in the pages that follow show in vivid detail how the reimbursement and regulatory frameworks shape nursing home care work, and how workers use emotional labor as a resource to construct a sense of dignity and meaning within the structural constraints of the workplaces.

Nursing home care work is a prototypical example of what sociologist Everett Hughes termed "dirty work." In this formulation, particular forms of labor are physically, socially, or morally devalued as disgusting, demeaning, and properly conducted out of the public eye.[16] Dirty work is delegated to groups who labor on society's behalf, doing necessary work that is then devalued and disowned by the society that has mandated such work be done. Although managers are to some extent shielded due to their status,[17] nursing home care work is stigmatized as something that nobody would seem to do willingly. Nursing assistants come to personify a set of repulsive tasks. Although nursing home care work includes food preparation, doing laundry, organizing activities, and completing paperwork, it is largely associated with the daily tasks done by nursing assistants such as assisting elderly individuals who have difficulty controlling their bowels or require help with bathing, dressing, and other routine daily activities that are necessary to live independently. In occupations such as these that are stigmatized and socially undesirable, workers tend to imbue work with meaning in a way that transcends the sum of its parts.[18] They also tend to have particularly strong and widely shared beliefs, values, and norms that mitigate the stigma of dirty work, although high turnover among the floor staff weakens the shared organizational culture compared to those of low turnover occupations.[19] The daily tasks of the job and the interactions staff have with coworkers, supervisors, residents, and family members are the raw materials workers use to make meaning out of their work.

Care work is more than a set of instrumental acts required to maintain the physical well-being of another individual. It is also an ethic comprising genuine concern, affection, emotions, and attentiveness to meeting the needs of a vulnerable person or group of people.[20] Nursing assistants and other floor staff draw from this broader conception of care, for residents but also about residents, to construct dignity in their dirty work.[21] Care work has an emotional component that cannot be adequately captured or regulated by markets.[22] It transcends a simple market exchange precisely because emotions permeate the relationship between the care provider and the care's recipient.[23]

The findings from the 2004 National Nursing Home Survey seem to validate the centrality of emotional attachments in paid care work. The survey asked a nationally representative sample of nursing assistants working in nursing homes about a range of work-related issues. When asked to choose from a list of reasons for staying at their current position, 99 percent of nursing assistants said they "enjoyed caring for others" and 97 percent responded "this kind of work feels good." As far as the next most common answers, 76 percent said they stayed at the job for coworkers, 69 percent said it was the flexible schedule, and 68 percent said they liked the location of the facility. Fewer than half said they stayed at the job because of the good pay and career advancement, and 35 percent reported they stayed for the benefits package.

Nursing home care workers have emotional attachments to the individuals they provide care to, even as those emotions are constrained by structural characteristics of long-term care.[24] Care work is devalued socially and materially because it is presumed to be a part of women's natural instinct to care for others.[25] It is something that women are seemingly supposed to do, with or without monetary remuneration. These assumptions about the value of care work, and the public policies that support them, bring personal notions of care into the public world of work.[26] For example, nursing home staff often relate to residents as fictive kin, or "like family."[27] Nursing home staff use the familial metaphors and rely on their own personal experiences with death to mentally process the strains of caring for dying people at their jobs.[28] The fictive kin relationship between staff and residents extends also to the families of residents, as each desire and appreciate close relationships with each other.[29]

Yet given the vertical hierarchy of nursing homes, perhaps it is not surprising that managers encourage staff to think of residents like family only to turn around and use those emotional ties to exploit these wage workers.[30] That is one way that the business of nursing homes undermines the social and emotional components of care work, even though emotional attachments between staff and residents are associated with higher work satisfaction and better health outcomes.[31] For example, Timothy Diamond's *Making Gray Gold*, a vivid ethnographic portrait of nursing homes, examined how the profit motive undermined opportunities for emotional closeness between staff and residents. Diamond's findings foreshadowed the takeover of long-term care by large for-profit corporations that have institutionalized chronic understaffing and work overload, at a huge cost to staff and residents.[32] As Francesca Cancian argued, "Organizations undermine care work by maximizing profits, creating hierarchical systems of authority that give little power to care workers, enforcing rigid procedures and rules, and promoting a system of values, incentives, and training that recognizes only medical knowledge."[33]

Emotions may be devalued in organizations, but they remain a central component of nursing home care work. Arlie Hochschild's *The Managed Heart: Commercialization of Human Feeling* is perhaps the most important contemporary analysis of emotions in the context of work. Hochschild showed how workers who provide a direct service to customers, a large and expanding sector of the workforce, align their inner emotions and outer displays of emotions (facial expressions, bodily gestures, etc.) with a set of rules, or norms, that are managed by organizations and driven by a logic of capitalist accumulation. Matching our emotions with what is expected and acceptable given the social context is a part of daily life.[34] Some emotion work happens effortlessly; in most settings, people know how they are expected to emote and do so accordingly without awareness of the normative expectations. However, the alignment of our emotions to the organizational boundaries of permissible and prohibited emotions, as often occurs in the context of work, represents a new form of labor exploitation that Hochschild called "emotional labor." Emotional labor happens when employees calibrate their inner emotions and outer displays of emotion with the "feeling rules" and "display rules" of a workplace. These rules are enforced by supervisors and occur within an institutional context that sets expectations over how workers are supposed to feel on the job. Emotional labor advances organizational goals at the expense of workers, who risk alienation from self when they repeatedly experience emotions that are not honestly felt. Hochschild combined the diverse perspectives of Erving Goffman, Charles Darwin, Sigmund Freud, and Karl Marx to argue that that emotional labor constitutes a form of labor exploitation unique to service work. When I began my field research,

I expected that managers would shape the emotional labor of workers in a manner broadly consistent with Hochschild's model. The boundaries that marked permissible and prohibited emotions would be clearly delineated and workers would be held accountable to those standards. I also expected a more tightly controlled emotional culture at the for-profit Golden Bay compared to the nonprofit Rolling Hills, given the fact that the construction of a positive, caring culture is a key dimension of competition among nursing homes. But that is not what I found. As I spent time with workers on the floor of the nursing home, it became increasingly clear that emotions were considerably more self-directed and useful for workers as they endured and even constructed a dignified view of their work and their reasons for staying on the job. A number of researchers, building off of Hochschild's foundation, have also shown the limits to the extent that organizations can control workers' emotional labor.[35]

The emotional labor that workers used, as a skill to build relationships that felt authentic and meaningful, is clearly an important part of nursing home care work. People from all walks of life struggle within the structural limitations of their workplaces to construct a sense of dignity at work.[36] Dignity is part of Enlightenment-era beliefs of individual autonomy, self-determination, reason, and virtue. It entails the ability to establish and maintain a fundamental feeling of self-worth and a self-evaluation of the worthiness and esteem inherent to a given behavior. This book highlights the role of emotions in the process of constructing dignity. Workers produced emotions, sometimes in ways consistent with organizational demands and sometimes not, but they consistently found in their emotions a resource to manage the strains of their work lives. They used emotions as rhetorical resources to cast their work, and their selves, in a positive light, reclaimed from the stigma of dirty work.

Outline of the Book

The book opens with a careful look at how reimbursement and regulatory structures shape nursing home care. Chapter 1 focuses on how staff managed Medicaid reimbursement, the largest contributor to nursing home revenues. The reimbursement system incentivizes the dependence and incapacity of residents, rather than encouraging independence and restorative care. In other words, Medicaid payment formulas promote the functional dependence of residents upon staff. The chapter details how nursing home staff tried to game the system without crossing the fraud line and the emotional conflict managers felt as this process unfolded. Chapter 2 examines the behind-the-scenes preparation by nursing homes for the annual health and safety inspection, the key tool used by CMS to monitor regulatory compliance. The inspections force nursing homes to maintain a baseline of safety for residents' health, but they also normalize structural problems such as chronic understaffing and work overload. Each nursing assistant was assigned to care for ten residents at the same time. Each nurse had twenty residents. These staffing ratios are consistent with the industry standard and were not considered problematic during the inspections, even though they caused a lot of problems for nursing assistants who struggled to do all the work that needed to get done without cutting corners here and there.

The first two chapters reveal the set of constraints and pressures that nursing home managers face from the reimbursement and regulatory structures. They were compelled to treat care work as a series of instrumental, reimbursable acts in a system that does not provide enough resources. Nursing home residents became the embodiment of those reimbursable acts. Chapter 3 builds on this analysis by showing how these constraints generated conflict between floor staff and managers, given the steep workplace hierarchies. The structural context of nursing home care work pulled floor workers and managers toward different sets of priorities; indeed, they often seemed to work in entirely different social worlds.[37] The concerns of the floor staff were pulled down to residents' daily needs while managers' interests were pulled up to the reimbursement and regulatory procedures, leading to different orientations and routine conflict toward the documentation that was critical for reimbursement and regulatory compliance.

Building off of this structural context, chapter 4 examines the consequences of practicing nursing home care in a way that is misaligned with the constraints of the reimbursement system. While the for-profit Golden Bay won awards for their solid financial performance, the nonprofit Rolling Hills edged to the brink of financial ruin. Rolling Hills' "first-come, first-served" admission policy, which did not discriminate against Medicaid recipients in favor of much more lucrative Medicare recipients—a key component of their nonprofit, altruistic orientation—caused a severe revenue crisis and ultimately led to Andy's termination. The story I tell here is not simply about Andy's personal failure, although it is surely that. It is also a story about the failure of nonprofit idealism and, more generally, about the failure of American social policy to develop an alternative to profit-driven nursing home care. It is, in this sense, a story about how and why nonprofits come to behave like for-profits but also about what is lost in that process. Chapter 5 extends the analysis in chapter 4, tracing the effects of the revenue crisis at Rolling Hills to their dietary department, including forced cuts to the budget for food and meal service. This chapter documents how the budgetary austerity directly harmed residents' quality of life and the morale of Rolling Hills' work force.

Given the structural context that constrains nursing home care, reducing care to a series of instrumental acts and turning residents into an embodiment of reimbursable activities, workers turned to matters they could seemingly control to make the work bearable. They concentrated on their caring, emotional attachments with residents. Chapter 6 shows how nursing home care workers used emotional labor as a skill, a symbolic resource, to enhance and provide a sense of dignity at work. At the same time, they used emotional labor to control unwanted resident behaviors. The chapter also shows how these processes sometimes broke down into unresolved conflict. Chapter 7 builds on this analysis by examining how nursing home care workers made attributions of agency or the lack of agency about residents in order to make sense of, and cope with, residents' behavior.

The concluding chapter 8 brings together the central themes of the book by connecting the experience of nursing home care workers to the experience of residents. The reimbursement and regulatory systems focus on a very narrow range of care that undermines residents' quality of life and staff morale in some really critical ways. The burgeoning "culture change movement" aims to improve the physical, social, and emotional environment of nursing homes, but there will be no significant cultural change without major structural changes. The United States faces a huge challenge in terms of how we are going to care for the aged over the next thirty years. We know that the number of people who will need long-term care is going to rise dramatically, as the baby boomers retire and life expectancy increases. Yet we have done very little to prepare for the increasing need for long-term care. We also know that there is going to be a steep increase in the number of people who will be working in occupations that take care of the elderly. Yet we have also done very little to make these jobs more attractive to people who might be good at nursing home care work but stay away because of the low pay and low prestige of these jobs. The fates of the individuals who need long-term care services and the people who provide those services are deeply connected. Both have suffered from neglect, and now is the time to illuminate the structures that shape those fates, before it is too late to do anything but cope in a broken, overwhelmed system.

1

Making the Most of Medicaid

Victoria burst through Andy's door and presented him, triumphantly, with a document full of names and numbers. As the Medicaid reimbursement coordinator for Rolling Hills, she had just completed her estimation of the reimbursement rate for all residents on Medicaid. She pointed out that the overall average reimbursement they would get from Medicaid went up, and, if her estimates were approved by the Medicaid auditors who would visit Rolling Hills in a few weeks, the nursing home was poised to increase the flow of revenue from Medicaid. Victoria was proud, indicating that her job was not simply to collect and ratify the documentation of care provided by floor staff; rather, it was to interpret the documentation in a way to obtain the most revenue from Medicaid, the health care insurance system for the poor and disabled, which is notorious among health care providers for low reimbursements compared to all other forms of payment. Delighted, Andy let loose a figurative, "I could just kiss you!" As they discussed final audit preparations, Lenny stopped in just to say hello on the way outside for his daily walk. A spry old man with gray hair hidden under a Red Sox cap, Lenny chatted with them for a moment, then strolled down the hallway and out the front door. Andy turned to me and quietly complained that Medicaid paid Rolling Hills only one hundred dollars a day to care for Lenny. Andy slowly reiterated "one hundred dollars a day," fully enunciating each syllable for dramatic effect. I asked how much a room costs for people who pay for nursing home care services out of their savings, and Victoria said that a "semiprivate," or shared, room cost two hundred thirty-six dollars per day. Andy turned toward me and snapped, "I should be charging more than that."

Nursing home managers push for the documentation of daily care that makes Medicaid residents look incapable and dependent because it increases their reimbursements. This runs counter to the policy framework enacted in the 1987 Nursing Home Reform Act, that nursing homes are to help residents be as independent as possible and work with residents through occupational, physical, and speech therapy to restore capabilities they may have lost. Medicaid incentives run in the opposite direction: if a nursing home succeeds in helping a resident achieve continence, or restores the ability to eat independently, and documents that achievement accurately, the facility receives fewer dollars to pay for that resident's care. Medicaid's narrow working definition of "care" as a series of discrete, instrumental, reimbursable acts of manual assistance undermines nursing homes' interest and ability to keep residents as independent as possible. In other words, Medicaid financially rewards dependence and incapacity. More acts of documented care mean more reimbursements.

Nursing home care workers, constrained by this set of rules they did not like, used emotional and rhetorical strategies within those constraints to feel content about their jobs. The reimbursement coordinators used a rhetoric of professionalism to frame their resistance to pressures by upper management to game the system. The state auditors, who inspected the documentation by hand at the nursing homes, used "jokes" to reinforce their power to control the flow of reimbursement dollars. Both sides jostled over the "fraud line," pushing their particular interpretation of the reimbursement rules without actually contesting the rules themselves or impugning the motives of the parties involved. This caused considerable tension but ultimately reflected the power of the state to define what counts as care, with considerable impacts for care work, care workers, and, of course, the residents.

The data for these arguments are drawn mostly from Golden Bay because I had extraordinary access to the process there. Not long after I began fieldwork, I was offered a small desk to use in their financial office, an offer that became quite valuable because I gained unexpected and unprecedented insight into the reimbursement process and the financial constraints and opportunities of the nursing home industry more generally. Instead of showing how they play out at the level of policy,[1] I examine how they operate on the ground as managers wrestle with these conflicting priorities. My uncommon access into the process at Golden Bay allowed me to show something that does not appear anywhere in the existing literature and that is worth a bit of asymmetry.

The Medicaid Reimbursement Process

Medicaid is the primary government health insurance program that pays for long-term care in nursing homes. The program is managed by the Centers for Medicare and Medicaid Services, a division of the U.S. Department of Health and Human Services.[2] Oversight is principally federal, but each state administers its own Medicaid program and establishes its own eligibility standards, scope of services, and reimbursement rates to health services organizations. Many beneficiaries become poor enough to qualify for the program after "spending down" their life savings paying for nursing home care on their own. The median cost of a shared room in a nursing home is two hundred seven dollars per day, about seventy-five thousand annually.[3] In both nursing homes, it was fairly common for newly admitted residents to start out paying the nursing home from their savings until they were poor enough to qualify for Medicaid. Then they were placed on Medicaid until they died. Government data indicate that the average length of stay in a nursing home is 835 days.[4] Although approximately 60 percent of nursing home residents are on Medicaid, Medicaid reimbursement accounts for only 40 percent of all nursing home revenue, indicating comparatively low reimbursement rates per beneficiary.[5] Managers may not have known those specific figures, but they routinely stated that Medicaid reimbursements were much too low to cover operational costs. They said that Medicaid beneficiaries were usually a net financial loss for nursing homes, a claim supported by empirical research.[6] Median Medicaid payment rates at Rolling Hills and Golden Bay were about one hundred eighty dollars per resident per day, less than what the facilities charged individuals who paid for care out of pocket, which was about two hundred thirty per day for a shared room and two hundred seventy for a private room.

With Medicaid residents' care being reimbursed at such low rates, nursing homes interpret documentation aggressively to get the most Medicaid reimbursements possible. What research on payment mechanisms for nursing home care has missed is that the policies and regulations that govern reimbursement are put into practice and given meaning at the level of interaction between nursing home care workers and state auditors. Medicaid reimbursement coordinators learn, in their interactions with state regulators, where the fraud line is and how to alter documentation to maximize revenues in ways that approach the fraud line without crossing over. The auditors are "street-level bureaucrats," representatives of government policy who are afforded considerable discretion in how those policies are applied.[7]

After a few months of observations at Rolling Hills, I spent some time watching work in the financial office, a large, sunny room shared by three managers across the hall from Andy's office. Victoria sat behind a large desk with papers and binders strewn around a computer monitor and keyboard. She processed all the paperwork required for Medicaid reimbursements. Victoria was a veteran staff member at Rolling Hills, and her colleagues respected that she stayed at the nursing home through a period of organizational transition that led the upper management of the small chain of nonprofit nursing homes to hire Andy as administrator and Joanne as the director of nursing. Victoria was pleased with their leadership and described Andy as "a little spacey, but he—you know, he knows what he's doing." She often brought her children to the facility when there was a special event, such as the annual National Nursing Home Week in mid-May. In addition to coordinating Medicaid reimbursement paperwork, she doubled as the wound care specialist for the facility, arriving early in the morning to examine and treat pressure ulcers, or bed sores, among residents.

I sat in the financial office and watched Victoria train a nurse who worked at another facility in the company and would be processing its Medicaid reimbursement. They reviewed the documentation required for reimbursement, especially the Management Minutes Questionnaire (MMQ) form that maps acts of daily care onto the amount of time the state estimates that care should take. Reimbursement rates are set according to this estimation. Victoria told her, "For someone who is totally dependent for bathing, you get twenty minutes per twenty-four hours." That meant that Medicaid paid facilities for twenty minutes of bathing care, regardless of how long it actually took to bathe a resident who was totally dependent on the staff for that "activity of daily living." For eating, Victoria explained, "If the resident is totally dependent, you get forty-five minutes" per day, not per meal. As Victoria spoke, her mildly sarcastic tone of voice gave away her feeling that care cannot be adequately quantified in such a one-size-fits-all manner, since resident needs change across time and space. Victoria's trainee interjected, "But that's not real," suggesting that the state's reimbursement for forty-five minutes of care to feed three meals a day to a resident who is totally dependent on staff misrepresents what actually happens during meals. Victoria continued to teach. She explained that for a resident whom the state says, based on the entirety of the documentation, required two hundred minutes of care per day the nursing home would be reimbursed $182 per day, and added, "That's horrible." The conversation repeatedly circled back to the state's unrealistic characterization of resident care and the seemingly low reimbursement dollars connected to those characterizations. For an incontinent resident, "You get forty-eight minutes for twenty-four hours of toileting," Victoria said. The other nurse replied, "That doesn't make any sense at all for responsible care." Then she joked sarcastically, "Sorry, I can't take you to the bathroom until tomorrow" because they had already provided forty-eight minutes of bathroom care today. The trainee continued, "They [the state] know it's not true," and Victoria declared, "Right!" Lesson learned. At one point they simply traded adjectives as they stared at the documents: "horrible," "dreadful," and finally "Reimbursement! That's disgusting." The reimbursement system undermines residents as individuals, turning them into the personification of reimbursable activities that are neatly measured and quantified for the state. The rules demanded that care workers regard residents as calculable revenue based on instrumental and documented acts of care.

Medicaid reimbursement to nursing homes in the state is not allocated according to how much time it actually takes to provide care. Rather, it is based on state estimates of how much time care should take.[8] Victoria and her counterpart at Golden Bay, Crystal, filled out the MMQ form after the nursing assistants had filled out "flow sheets" that document the daily amount of care provided and nurses had completed their monthly summaries of the flow sheets. The MMQ is a fairly straightforward, one-page document with twenty-four types of care provided including bathing, dressing, eating, and so forth. For example, the section to document the assistance required to dress residents looks like this:

1. 4. Dressing
2. C1/S0—independent/restorative program
3. C2/S30—assist
4. C3/S30—totally dependent
5. C4/S0—socks and shoes only
6. C5/S0—nonambulatory Code = _____ Score = _____

The C stands for the code and S is the score, or the number of minutes the state determined such care should take and reimburses for. The same level of assistance must be marked on the nursing assistant's flow sheet for at least fifteen days of the "money month" (even if the money month is February). It is completed once every six months for each resident on Medicaid and submitted to the state, a process that staff members called the "turnaround." Several weeks later, auditors from the state Department of Public Health arrived to inspect the documentation. In principle, the audits are unannounced, but in practice the auditors notified the facility several days before the inspection began. Once the documentation passes the eyes of the state auditors, who are empowered to lower reimbursements at their discretion, the reimbursement rate for the prospective six months is determined.

Medicaid reimbursements ranged from eighty-seven to just over two hundred dollars per day. It is confusing that the state Medicaid program determines reimbursement rates based upon ten "case mix categories" determined by the number of minutes total, which are subsequently mapped onto six different "payment categories." For example, case mix category L covers 110.1 to 140 minutes of care per day and category M spans 141.1 to 170. Despite the different categories (and up to 60 minutes more care daily) the reimbursement amount was the same, $158 per day for the prospective six months at Golden Bay, slightly less at Rolling Hills.[9]

Medicaid residents like Lenny, mentioned at the beginning of this chapter, whose care was reimbursed for less than thirty minutes of measured care per day, paid the least, eighty-seven dollars per day. These are people who can do most things independently. Victoria explained that residents like Lenny are not good for the finances, but they are important for staff morale because they can carry on routine conversations. But those conversations came at a price. As Lucy, the director of nursing at Golden Bay, declared, "I mean there are residents in this building that we're only getting eighty-seven dollars a day. Eighty-seven dollars a day doesn't pay for anything. It does not pay for anything. I mean, it's basically free care."

Making the Most of Medicaid

The corporate management at both nursing homes closely monitored the Medicaid reimbursement coordinators, especially as the audits approached. Victoria at Rolling Hills stated that after she finished preparing for the audit, "My corporate leader, whatever you want to call her, comes out after I've done it and goes through every chart herself to make sure she can't find something more that I didn't find. So essentially they redo what I've just done, looking for more." This tight supervision also occurred at Golden Bay, a process I was allowed to observe.

Crystal, the Medicaid reimbursement coordinator at Golden Bay, spent her entire two-decade nursing career in long-term care and had held a variety of positions at different facilities, large and small, for-profit and nonprofit. This was her first "money position," as she called it, and with good reason. The administrator of the facility, Cynthia, occasionally introduced Crystal to others with the preface, meant only partially in jest, "The financial health of the building rides on her shoulders." Despite all the paperwork, she "loved" the facility and referred to her position as the best job she had ever had. Her large desk was adorned with photos of her children, a little pile of gemstones, and stacks of Medicaid-related paperwork and binders. At lunch one or two of her colleagues would often stop by to chat and coordinate takeout lunch orders from local restaurants.

A few weeks before the Medicaid audit at Golden Bay, I walked into the financial office to set down my backpack next to the small desk I had provided, but Paulette was sitting there. Paulette was Crystal's supervisor at the company's regional headquarters more than one hundred miles away, and she came to Golden Bay to review the Medicaid paperwork before the audit. Throughout the tedious review of the documentation, Paulette noted any discrepancies between forms. These inconsistencies in the documentation could be justification to deny the nursing home reimbursement for care they had done but recorded the wrong way. Paulette claimed that the nursing home had the right to reimbursement for care performed even when the documentation as originally written was not entirely consistent with the notation system that auditors required. She advised Crystal to revise documentation to be consistent with those specifications. For example, dementia unit nursing assistants documented that residents with dysphagia (difficulty swallowing) ate independently. "That's a problem," Paulette noted. Crystal said that the nursing assistants monitored eating but did not document it. "I've talked to the unit manager," Crystal explained. "I've left notes for them. It's a locked unit, so they are all supervised and they need to document that." This was one of Crystal's pet points. She said that all residents on the dementia unit, as well as those on the other units who ate in the dayrooms and the main dining room, should be documented as "continually supervised" for eating.

Documenting these residents as "continually supervised" would considerably boost reimbursement compared to documenting them as eating "independently." Crystal explained that nursing assistants do many forms of daily care that they take for granted and thus do not document when in fact the nursing home deserved to be reimbursed for these "invisible" forms of care. Paulette reiterated the "if it isn't documented, it didn't happen" rhetoric that is pervasive in bureaucracies and suggested that Crystal play off staff members' emotions to make sure the residents are supervised: "Explain to them what dysphagia is," Paulette said, "and then say, 'if it was your mother who had dysphagia and choked, you'd want someone to be supervising her.'" Crystal would follow up with the nursing assistants about the documentation of mealtime supervision.

Later in the day, Paulette noticed another inconsistency that she worried could lead to a denied reimbursement claim. One resident's care plan stated that she was "totally dependent" on staff for transfers (from the bed to the wheelchair to the bathroom and back). The daytime staff noted that two nursing assistants did the transfer, but the nighttime staff documented that only one nursing assistant transferred the person. Paulette said it looked strange: "Unless they are just a bag of bones, anyone who is totally dependent is a two-assist for transfers." Paulette continued that residents could be injured during one-assist transfers, but perhaps the nursing assistants were at even greater risk of injury. The Bureau of Labor Statistics reports that nursing assistants have some of the highest nonfatal injury and illness rates of all occupations.[10] Lifting and moving residents, often in cramped bathrooms and bedrooms, are leading sources of injuries among nursing home care workers, who report in excess of two hundred thousand annual cases of work-related back pain.[11] Crystal continued to defend the care that nursing assistants provided and said the problem was with their documentation habits. "I have a feeling they are doing the right thing, but not documenting correctly," she said. Crystal's belief that care was not documented even though it was provided justified the revision to documentation in a way that raised reimbursements without crossing, in her view, the fraud line. If the nursing assistants were giving care that was simply not documented correctly, then Crystal was correcting what amounted to a clerical error.

All parties involved knew there was more to reimbursement than the simple collection and ratification of documentation. This was Crystal's first audit, and she was learning what the upper management expected. Days before the audit commenced, she received a call from Paulette to alert her that Medicaid auditors would no longer allow nursing homes to claim reimbursement for repositioning residents who are unable to reposition independently due to a cognitive impairment (routine repositioning of residents prevents pressure ulcers). Of course, the nursing assistants would continue to reposition cognitively impaired residents, but the nursing home could no longer bill Medicaid for the care. After Crystal got off the phone, she and I walked to the Dementia Unit, where virtually all the residents are on Medicaid.[12] She scanned medical charts to ensure that the facility would not lose potential Medicaid money because of how repositioning was documented. Flipping through the charts quickly, she stopped midway through one of them. She slid the signed and dated nursing summary out of its dust jacket and almost put her pen to the paper before she paused to ask a nurse for a black pen, rather than the blue one she held in her hand. With the correct pen, she made a few quick notations to document that staff repositioned this individual for reasons unrelated to the dementia, to which it was actually related. Crystal explained that the state makes it intentionally difficult for nursing homes to be paid fairly for their services, and she felt justified to claim as many reimbursements as she could. Her job, and in a sense everyone else's at Golden Bay, hinged on her ability to make the most of Medicaid reimbursement in a way that could be justified given the inherent ambiguities in the process. There will always be ambiguity in documentation and the meaning of care because in real life human beings do not act according to the categories constructed by any system, let alone a medical reimbursement system. Ultimately it was the state auditors who resolved the ambiguities in the system.

The Audit

Although Crystal was nervous about her first audit, she encouraged me to observe the process and even called Betty, the lead auditor, on my behalf to seek her permission. I thought there was no way Betty would allow it, but Crystal said that Betty was "very educational," and after a brief explanation of my project she allowed it. A few days later, I arrived at Golden Bay at eight o'clock in the morning, about a half hour before the auditors, Betty and Debby, arrived. I walked through the double doors and past the receptionist into the foyer. I continued through the main hallway to the financial office. Crystal had prepared coffee, tea, and pastries in the adjacent conference room where the state auditors would set up camp. The conference room at Golden Bay, like the one at Rolling Hills, looked a lot like an outdated household dining room, with a brass chandelier, flowery wallpaper on the walls, and framed, nondescript artwork.

Debby and Betty arrived at eight thirty sharp. "Oh, this is your first audit?" Debby asked Crystal. "I hope we don't make you cry! Or quit!" Debby and Betty, RNs with decades of combined years of nursing home experience, teased Crystal throughout the two-day audit. The auditors were in a unique position that allowed them to grasp the pressures that managers were under to game the system. Yet they also sympathized with the managers, even as they acted as the embodied extensions of the state. Seasoned veterans, they knew what it was like on both sides of the regulations.

Debby and Betty let me sit with them in the conference room. They crafted identities as tough yet understanding auditors, and they seemed to enjoy telling me stories of making nurses cry or walk off the job. One of them even boasted that her tires had been slashed in a nursing home parking lot. I sat next to Debby, and they sat across from each other, as they scrutinized the documentation written by nursing assistants and nurses and organized by Crystal. This was a tedious process; they reviewed by hand all the germane documentation for every Medicaid resident. Betty explained that they used to review only a random sample of charts to calculate reimbursement rates, but at some point years ago the regulations were tightened and now they were required to review all residents' medical charts. When the supportive documentation did not reach the fifteen-day threshold to justify reimbursement, Betty looked at Crystal over her reading glasses and said simply, as if she was a machine, "It does not compute."

As we sat amid medical charts, piles of paper, and empty coffee cups, Betty and Debby seemed happy to have someone there who wanted to learn about their work. "Most homes are truthful, but sometimes people push the truth to fraud," Debby said. She turned to her colleague Betty, and coyly asked a leading question, "We don't have any that go too far, do we?" The quieter of the two, Betty said nothing but raised her eyebrow and smirked. Moments later, Betty turned to me and declared, "There's a lot more fraud than you think." She added, "We get really suspicious when we see perfect documentation, where everything is perfectly clean and matching. Or the way they will write a 2 straight down the CNA flow sheet.[13] It's like, you know, *has the ink dried yet on this flow sheet* [spoken as she waved a piece of paper in the air]?" When Betty gets suspicious about the accuracy of the documentation she will observe the unit and may ask residents directly about their care. If the documentation is not corroborated by her observations, she will deny the reimbursement claim.

Neither Betty nor Debby blamed the reimbursement coordinators themselves for crossing the fraud line; in fact, they said that the managers will sometimes confide in them about the pressures they face from upper management to alter documentation. Betty told me of a coordinator who discovered that her MMQ forms had been replaced by new ones written by her director of nursing, who forged the coordinator's signature. But the auditors did not blame the managers so much as they blamed the structure of the health care system. Betty said, "There is a lot of money in nursing care. Why do you think all these corporations are buying them up?" She added, "The pressure on the nurses is coming from above, they are trying to squeeze every penny they can out of Medicaid." For good measure, Betty added, "The corporate regional people are making lots of money, and it is not filtering down to the people who need it." I said it seemed like there was a lot of pressure on the reimbursement coordinators to navigate a vague boundary between getting as much Medicaid money as they can without overstepping into fraud, and I suggested that "they're damned if they do, and damned if they don't." If they do push on the boundary they risk a fraud accusation and potential investigation by the state; if they do not, they risk leaving Medicaid money on the table and getting into trouble at work.

The reimbursement coordinators experienced these tensions in their dealings up the organizational hierarchy with corporate management and the state, but they also experienced them down the organizational hierarchy as they requested that floor staff revise documentation already done or change their future documentation practices. For example, the issue of whether residents ate meals continually supervised or independently generated conflict between nurse managers and floor staff. Crystal saw it as considerable lost revenue, evident in the large, laminated signs she taped next to the Care-Tracker documentation kiosks that read, "every resident should be documented as supervised for their meals." This was one of many daily reimbursable acts of care that Crystal said the floor staff took for granted and thus did not document. She contended, "Just because the resident puts a spoon into their mouths does not mean they are independent." The staff watched residents to ensure that they ate, documented how much they ate, and made sure that they ate safely, all of which, Crystal argued, entitled the nursing home to reimbursement money.

The signs by the kiosks were impossible to miss, yet nursing assistants continued to document, and nurses continued to ratify, that residents ate independently. I shadowed Crystal as she tracked down staff members to request that they sign revised forms that showed supervised eating. We took the elevator upstairs and walked behind the nursing station of the rehabilitation unit. With their backs turned to the hallway, Crystal stood next to Carissa, a clinically experienced nurse with management experience, and asked her to sign a nursing summary Crystal authored. Carissa perused the document and asked, "Well where's the CNA documentation saying [eating is] supervised?" Crystal said, "Well, I still have to change that." Carissa refused to sign. She told Crystal, "I know corporate wants to make money, I totally understand that, but it's my license and I can't put my signature on this without seeing the documentation first." Carissa snickered sarcastically and continued, "Most of these people aren't supervised when they are eating; they are in a room with forty residents. Just because a CNA is in the room, that doesn't mean they are being supervised." Crystal appeared a tad discouraged as we rode the elevator back down, and concluded with a depleted sigh, "She's right."

The audit vindicated Carissa. Debby and Betty denied the claims for supervised eating. Crystal protested, "But everyone on the dementia unit is supervised." Debby grumbled, made eye contact with me, and said in a stern, authoritative tone, "Just because you're eyeballing them once in a while does not indicate continual supervision. It does not compute." She added, "There's nothing you can do about it now, just take this as a learning experience." Crystal argued that everyone on the unit was supervised simply because a nurse or nursing assistant was in the same room as the residents. The concept of "supervision," initially left to the interpretation of nursing staff, was trumped by the auditors' narrower interpretation. They claimed that residents needed to be observed personally during meals to assist with eating and prevent choking. There is simply not enough staff to provide that level of care. Ultimately the regulatory language that appears at first glance to be clear and unequivocal turns out to be subject to an interpretive process shaped by position within the organizational structure of nursing home care.

At this point, Crystal became concerned, even paranoid, that the auditors were suspicious of her. Throughout the audit she repeatedly popped her head into the conference room and asked, "So, things still going okay in here?" Debby laughed heartily and joked, "It's only been five minutes since you last asked. If you ask again you'll invoke Murphy's Law." Crystal showed her anxiety and jumped to conclusions, "What, you'll start getting suspicious?" And Debby said, "No, it will start to go downhill" and teased her in the tone of a game show host, "Oh, I'm going to find a lot to take away on the next one, big money, big money!"

There was a predictable arc to these interactions: when Debby and Betty found something that did not compute, Crystal inquired if it lowered the reimbursement rate, and the auditors teased Crystal with obvious exaggerations about lost money. They used humor to remind Crystal of their authority to deny reimbursement claims at their discretion. At one point, for example, they found a problem with the documentation for seizure control. Betty told Crystal, "If everyone in the facility knows how to use the magnet then it is no longer a skilled observation."[14] She remembered from the previous audit that even the housekeepers were trained to use the magnet. Crystal cut to the chase: "Is this a money thing?" No. "Oh, thank God," Crystal said, and Debby kidded with a smile, "It's three thousand dollars a day and it's coming out of your paycheck!"

The auditors' use of humor and jokes only reinforced the ways nursing home care was reduced to a disembodied set of reimbursable activities. They also reinforced the power imbalance in the interaction. There is a long history of using humor to highlight and clarify how inequality shapes the organization of daily life.[15] The "jokes" are the type of jokes that someone in power uses to assert authority over someone else. The auditors used jokes as a mechanism to reinforce their authority in a palatable way. The auditors and nursing home managers are in a unique place because they are all RNs and share the same occupational training, background, and prestige. In these senses they are on the same level. But at the same time there is a structural imbalance to the interaction because the auditors have the power to deny reimbursements. The auditors let Crystal know that even though they are all nurses, they are not equal parties to the interaction.

Betty and Debby examined the repositioning documentation as Crystal walked into the conference room. Betty asked, "Why is there only documentation for repositioning on the seven to three shift? What happens after three to seven a.m.? At three in the afternoon, where is she? And at four, five, six? Because you can't routinely be taking positioning on all these folks who are limited assist. You have to be really careful about that. It just does not compute." Crystal asked, "Is there any way to salvage this?" Betty responded, simply, "No." Crystal took a risk and asked, "Well, could I go have the nurse put in the information?" Debby rebutted sharply, "No! Don't even talk like that!" Crystal murmured "okay," chuckled nervously, then turned around and walked out of the conference room. Debby turned to me and said, "That's what drives me crazy. This leaves such a sour taste in my mouth that people are doing it who you'd never think are doing it."

Crystal broke the unspoken rules of the interaction. It was firmly on the wrong side of the fraud line to suggest altering documentation during the audit. When I caught up to Crystal in the hallway, she bawled dramatically, "Jason I can't take it! I feel like I'm on trial!" Betty and Debby expected nursing homes to test the rules, and Crystal expected the auditors to take away as many claims as they could. But Crystal had brazenly tested whether or not the auditors would apply the rules when challenged explicitly. Although the auditors at some moments used their authority to give Crystal the benefit of the doubt, especially because it was her first audit, they were not about to give her permission to break the rules.

Betty and Debby allowed me to observe the exit meeting, when they explained the findings of the audit to Crystal and the nursing home's billing manager. Debby joked that the billing manager might need some Kleenex and moved the box of tissues right in front of him. In keeping with the theme, Betty teased, "We took away the thirty million!" referring to the large sums of money that hinged on reimbursement. The billing manager was not amused. Not one for humor, he turned to me and deadpanned, "That's because they work on commission." Debby replied defensively, "We don't work on commission! People just think we do."

Debby delivered the news. Out of one hundred charts reviewed, they made sixteen changes in the amount of reimbursable minutes, nine of which resulted in a money loss. Afterward, Debby told me these numbers were about average for a facility of this size. Debby went through each change individually, described the original documentation, including what did not compute and the lower reimbursement category based on their findings. As the exit interview concluded, Betty teased, "See, that wasn't so bad!" And Debby added, "You didn't even need a Kleenex!" Crystal was unsure what to think, but her colleagues and the administrator congratulated her on a job well done, especially since the previous audit of the nursing home's Medicaid documentation included twice as many monetary losses.

Nursing homes could provide care that promotes independence and the restoration of lost abilities, but Medicaid's payment structure works the opposite way. It promotes dependence on staff-assisted care, as nursing homes are reimbursed more when residents are fully dependent on them than when they are independent. If a nursing home restores the ability of a stroke survivor to walk without staff assistance, the reimbursement dollars go down, not up. Few know this better than the Medicaid reimbursement coordinators. At a staff meeting at Rolling Hills, after the speech pathologist announced that a resident's condition had improved to the point that she could eat independently, Victoria snickered, "Oh great, we've done such a good job that we get paid less!" because the staff no longer assisted her as she ate. At Golden Bay, Crystal explained to me, "I always say that their loss is our gain." She meant that residents' physical decline is in the financial interest of the nursing home because staff must provide more assistance with residents' activities of daily living.

Put differently, this explains why managers look the other way when nursing assistants chart care that wasn't actually done—a consistent finding in the ethnographic literature on nursing homes.[16] From the perspective of reimbursement, documenting care that was not done is not a problem; instead, what is truly problematic for nursing home managers, as Crystal pointed out again and again, is *care that was given but not documented* because it cannot be reimbursed. Furthermore, Medicaid reimbursement formulas mean that time spent providing social or emotional support, a crucial failing of the nursing home industry as a whole, is invisible and not reimbursable.

Auditing Emotions

The Medicaid audits are the key piece of the overall reimbursement process, in which a dynamic and ever-changing flow of care practices are transformed into a discrete set of reimbursable activities. Residents come to embody those activities and become a site of revenue generation. This shapes nursing home financing, the character of care work, and the experience of care for the residents, but it also shapes how staff members experience and make meaning of their work. The reimbursement process made the staff feel bad about their jobs. Constrained within a system they did not like, they used a rhetoric of professionalism to make themselves feel better about what they were doing. People tend to use rhetorical strategies to neutralize or justify the impact of potentially stigmatizing behaviors.[17] Previous research has looked at the neutralization techniques of nursing home care workers who knowingly overcharge Medicare and Medicaid.[18] Such "vocabularies of motive" are intended to minimize the negative impact, symbolic or material, of questionable documentation practices on the self-concept of nursing home care workers.[19] Crystal and Victoria made attributions of intent toward self and others involved in the process, relying on a rhetoric of professionalism to resist demands from those above them to massage the documentation for higher reimbursements.

For example, after Golden Bay's audit, I noticed a small sign on Crystal's desk. It was handwritten and attached with a paper clip to a photo of her children. It read, in colored block letters, simply, "integrity." She told me about that sign in our interview:

> CRYSTAL: I did what I had to do [for the audit]. I'm not sure I feel entirely
>   good about it, which is why I have that little integrity sign on my desk
>   now, which is a reminder that that's exactly where I came from.
> JASON: Why do you feel like in the last audit—?
> CRYSTAL: Yeah. I feel like I really stretched the limits. I feel like I asked for
>   things that I'm not entirely convinced of.
> JASON: And did that bother you?
> CRYSTAL: Terribly. Yeah. It really bothered me. It really bothered me when
>   we had points taken away. We lost sixty dollars a day on a particular
>   person because I had overreached based on the "blitz" [review] we did
>   with Paulette who looked through all the care plans and on paper it
>   seemed like the person might have been more needy then she actually
>   is in her day-to-day life. So I based my [documentation] on a need that
>   really doesn't play out in her day-to-day life and the auditor knew that
>   patient from years ago and she knew darn well that that person wasn't
>   incontinent to the degree I said. And didn't need the toileting help that
>   I said that they needed.

Crystal explained that her corporate supervisor, Paulette, pushed her to "no holds barred, go for the money." Crystal operated within this structure and did not like how it shaped her work. To resolve this dilemma, she ascribed agency to others and the interests they represented in selective ways that allowed her to reclaim a self that stood apart from the reimbursement process. Crystal said the corporate office cared only about the bottom line, the auditors represented the state that made reimbursement intentionally difficult, and she was something of a pawn in the process, left with hurt feelings and conceptions of self that bordered on dishonorable. Crystal pushed back against the structure of nursing home care with a rhetoric of professionalism—she explained, "It's my license on the line" and that her supervisors had the legal safety of not being the one required to sign the forms. The integrity sign on her desk, clipped to a picture of her children, was a call to herself not to be a pawn in the process and instead assert agency to resist the reimbursement pressures.

Victoria at Rolling Hills, like Crystal at Golden Bay, also felt bad about the audit process because of the ways it shaped what she had to do on the job. During the Rolling Hills audit, I caught up with Victoria in the break room. Throughout a career in nursing home care, she had experienced many audits and had a good working relationship with Debby and Betty, whom she described as "really fair" and even "cool." But she was concerned. As she stood next to the vending machines with a soda in her hand, she confided, "[Corporate] made me claim stuff that Debby is going to take away. I did it this time for them but I won't do it again. *It's my license at stake.*" Prior to the audit, her corporate supervisor came to the facility, reviewed documentation, and asked her to write new MMQs to claim a higher reimbursement rate than the originals declared. Victoria knew that the claims she was asked to make were not fully justified by the documentation, and, much like Crystal, she relied on a professional and legal framework to register her concerns. In my interview with Victoria several weeks later, I asked about the audit. She explained, "I do feel, especially around the time of the turnaround, that the corporate entity wants a lot more out of it than there is. I mean, you know, they really want me trying to take stuff that really ain't there. Trying to—you know; make people look dependent that aren't. I won't do that. I mean, they really try to stretch and pull whatever minutes they can out of the MMQ. And I understand where they're coming from, too, but you know, I can't." Andy praised her in a staff meeting for pushing the average Medicaid reimbursement up to $182 per day, but that reward went only so far. Victoria said she could not make people look more dependent than they really were, but alas she had little say in the matter beyond the rhetorical strategy and emotional labor that smoothed out whatever dissonance the process generated. The entire audit process undermined the notion that high-quality care for the elderly was the primary goal of nursing home care. It seemed to reduce care to a cold, calculated transaction. It turned residents into the embodiment of reimbursable activities and turned staff into instruments of a greedy system.

2

Staging the Inspections

I sat on the floor of the financial office at Rolling Hills as the managers filed in for a hastily scheduled meeting. Just a few hours earlier, inspectors from the Department of Public Health had arrived, unannounced, to conduct their annual health and safety inspection. The mood felt tense; the managers spent months preparing for this moment that had finally arrived. Andy, the administrator, was quietly optimistic that the inspection would go well. But he was also nervous that the inspectors might find something that would cause them to widen the scope of the survey. Andy may have taken his performance cues from sports, because as he entered the room clutching a clipboard, he had the look of a coach ready to prepare his team before a big game. Andy told the group that he had given the inspectors a tour of the facility this morning. Tomorrow they would begin "tearing through units in a quick fashion," he said, "which probably works to our advantage." Andy instructed them how to behave toward the state inspectors. He told them they needed to be careful in what they said and how they reacted to the inspectors' questions or requests. "I am giving you direction on what I want your demeanor to be," he explained. "Be normal. Be calm. When pressure arises, step outside yourself and stay calm." Andy was coaching their emotions. He continued, "We've had some hiccups, some call outs," but he insisted that they must remain calm and work hard. Two nursing assistants who worked the day shift had called in sick. The scheduler was calling nursing assistants who had the day off to offer them cash bonuses if they would come in to work. Joanne, the director of nursing, praised the managers, "Keep doing what you're doing, nice job." "We look good in the kitchen," Andy said. The kitchen was a key point of concern for Andy because the nursing home had, in the last inspection, been cited for several violations related to food storage and unsanitary conditions. Andy told Flo, the dietary manager, that one of the inspectors told him that the kitchen "looked much better." He continued, "Whatever she told you about, fix it, and you're all set." Andy reported that the inspectors found no "environmental red flags" on the units, and reminded them, "The eye on the prize is a busy, productive two days. Sometime there will be a heightened concern, it could be that a DNR [do not resuscitate order] is not in place, or there's something with a wound, but we all need to be ready and prepared." Andy encouraged them to "grind like crazy! The more we work together, the better shape we're in!"

Andy's speech to his "team," as he often referred to the managers, is a classic example of what sociologist Erving Goffman called "backstage" talk. In this chapter I draw from the dramaturgical perspective Goffman developed in his first and most well-known book, *The Presentation of Self in Everyday Life*. When individuals enter into an interaction, Goffman argued, they attempt to control the impressions they give off to others by carefully managing what they say, how they look, and the immediate social context around them. Put simply, Goffman saw a connection between how people present themselves and a theatrical performance, and he drew from metaphors of the stage to elucidate his central concepts. Goffman's work implies that people construct and sustain identities in face-to-face interactions, particularly interactions structured "within the physical confines of a building or plant." He often referred to medical settings in the anecdotes he used to support his premises.[1]

Following Goffman, I refer to conversations that occurred outside the view of state inspectors as "backstage" interactions and the main interactions and behaviors that occur in front of inspectors as "frontstage" interactions.[2] The staff's frontstage behavior is intended for the state inspectors, who are, in Goffman's lingo, the "audience." The audience is not simply a passive observer; rather, the audience implicitly endorses the authenticity of the act. Backstage, the actors prepare for the performance and also have more latitude to express thoughts and actions that contradict the impression they want to give off in the frontstage interactions. My vantage point as a participant-observer allowed me unique access to view frontstage performances as well as the backstage area where staff met privately. The nursing homes' managers took the inspections extraordinarily seriously and were fearful of the consequences of a bad outcome. An inspection that revealed a high number of regulatory deficiencies could dramatically worsen their financial standing. The Center for Medicare and Medicaid Services (CMS) releases inspection results to the public and encourages prospective customers to use them as a guide to choosing a nursing home. But there was also the matter of general reputation. Bad inspection results could attract unwanted and unfavorable media attention, closer scrutiny from the state, and micromanagement from corporate supervisors. The inspection results had material and social consequences for the nursing homes so that managers feared just thinking about them.

Long-term care is a heavily regulated industry. Yet the enforcement of those regulations implicitly normalizes a set of structural problems that generate a wide range of other issues.[3] For example, chronic understaffing is an industry-wide practice in nursing homes, with one nursing assistant typically assigned to ten residents and one nurse assigned to twenty residents. Understaffing in nursing homes extends beyond the nursing units; dietary, activities, and maintenance services occur with skeleton crews of low-wage and often part-time staff. During the inspections, nursing homes avoid the realities of understaffing by having managers work alongside nursing assistants passing out lunch trays, feeding residents, and performing other tasks typically done by low-wage floor staff. Managers worked on the floor of the nursing home to provide adequate staff to meet the residents' needs, particularly at mealtimes. The inspectors validated these performances, even though they know that managers do not typically do the work of nursing assistants. In this sense, the inspections normalize the chronic understaffing that characterizes nursing home care across the country. The inspections focus on a wide range of issues related to nursing home quality, but they also turn a blind eye to the problem that underlies so many others, understaffing and work overload.[4]

The Inspection Process

The annual health and safety inspection is the most critical tool of regulatory control over nursing homes. Consistent with regulations set forth in the Nursing Home Reform Act of 1987, all states must conduct unannounced inspections on nursing homes on an annual basis. Regulations are federally based, but the states manage enforcement. Nursing homes must meet the minimum requirements of these regulatory standards. The inspectors may issue a deficiency citation if they find something that is not compliant with regulations. Depending on the nature of the deficiency, CMS can take a variety of actions. For example, they may assess a fine, deny Medicaid and Medicare reimbursement to the nursing home, assign a temporary administrator, or install a state monitor. The extent of the penalty is determined by how much harm to residents was caused, or could be caused, by that particular violation. After the inspection, the nursing home must write and implement a "plan of correction" to remediate any deficiencies found during the inspection. The state must certify the soundness of the correction before clearing the nursing home until the next inspection the following year.

The inspections that enforce the regulations concern a wide range of areas, including proper handling of medication, protecting residents from physical or mental abuse and inadequate care, and ensuring the safe storage and preparation of food. Inspectors review the residents' clinical records, interview some residents and family members about their life in the nursing home, and interview caregivers and administrative staff. They also review 10 percent of residents' medical charts, chosen randomly. The inspectors have wide discretion to expand their inspection, which typically lasts three or four days.

Focusing on these things is not without its benefits, but it also implicitly accepts the understaffing problem endemic to nursing home care. There is simply not enough staff on shift for all the assigned work to be completed, forcing staff members to cut corners and then cover them up before the inspections. The long-term consequences of understaffing underscored much of the conflict I observed at the nursing homes. The Medicaid reimbursement issues I discussed in the previous chapter may not be such a problem if the facilities were adequately staffed to meet residents' needs while also completing documentation. Furthermore, just as the emphasis on care as reimbursable instrumental acts structures the work environment, the implicit acceptance of low staffing levels by CMS also structures the work environment.

In the period when this research was conducted, more than 90 percent of nursing homes were cited for regulatory violations in their annual health and safety inspection.[5] For-profit nursing homes averaged 7.6 deficiencies, more than nonprofits, which averaged 5.7. Government-owned facilities averaged 6.3 deficiencies. Rolling Hills had an above average number of regulatory violations for several consecutive inspections prior to Andy's arrival. In addition to a handful of relatively minor infractions, they were cited several times for serious regulatory violations that put residents in danger or in some cases were found to have caused actual harm. It was around that time that several nurse-managers quit and the nursing home went through a turbulent period of staff turnover. When Andy was hired Rolling Hills was, in his words, "a mess." He fired the director of nursing and in her place hired Joanne Lane, whom he said had a stellar reputation with the state nursing home inspectors. Joanne had an encyclopedic knowledge of the regulations and a nononsense demeanor. Andy once joked to me that when Joanne walked down the halls the nursing assistants scurried into the resident rooms to stay on her good side.

At the time of my research, the average number of deficiencies across the region was five, with a range of zero to thirty-three. Severe infractions were known as "G-level" or "G-tags," which indicated actual harm was caused to at least a few residents. For example, if a resident was injured in a fall and the state inspectors conclude that the staff did not appropriately follow the plans in place to prevent a fall, the facility will likely be served with a G-level violation that requires the facility to pay a fine and submit a plan of correction to satisfy state inspectors that the violation will not be repeated. A less severe infraction, such as food served at too low of a temperature, may come with a D-level violation that is unlikely to trigger a fine, although the facility still needs to develop a plan of correction to fix the problem. Managers said that inspectors seemed to prioritize certain areas of focus that changed annually. They told me that in speaking to their colleagues at recently inspected nursing homes, CMS was particularly focused on disaster planning because of Hurricane Katrina in 2005.[6]

The inspections, which staff referred to as "surveys," must be conducted between nine and fifteen months after the preceding survey, but CMS may conduct them more frequently at their discretion. The six-month window kept the managers at Rolling Hills and Golden Bay in a kind of frenzied anticipation. From the day the window opened until the day of the survey, the nursing homes administrators and directors of nursing reminded the staff to make sure all their documentation was in order because CMS could walk through the front door at any moment. The survey window implicitly monitored behavior even without the presence of inspectors because the anxiety of an unanticipated arrival by CMS was real and motivational.

The nursing home managers were held responsible for much of the backstage preparation work for the survey. The administrators and directors of nursing used emotional appeals, generating fear and anxiety among the managers about the inspections, frequently reminding them that the state could arrive at any moment. After the inspection window opened, they warned managers repeatedly to be on high alert for the state surveyors. One manager asked Joanne if she would be notified when the state arrived and Joanne snickered, "Oh yes, you'll be notified!" and warned that the state has been known to conduct inspections at night and over weekends. Another manager mimicked the urgent tone of the director of nursing in the run-up to the survey: "This needs to be done. That needs to be done. Do it. Do it. Do it. Do it. Do it." She continued, speaking as herself, "And you know—yeah, okay. Cool. I need that leadership. But you know, we're human beings. Let's figure out how we can do this and not be like overly stressed here." She described the stress she feels when the survey window opens, "It's like every night, before I go to bed my stomach starts churning. Every day when I wake up, I start thinking—oh, are they coming in today?" The looming inspections generated fear and anxiety, and the top leadership in the nursing homes used those feelings as a rhetorical tool to motivate the managers to prepare for the surveys.

In addition to the anxiety and the fear of the state inspections, managers also described feelings of having their work misunderstood by a process that was focused on the technical parts of nursing home care rather than the social and emotional components. Patricia, the staff educator at Golden Bay, said that she tells new employees during their training period, "I think it's a good thing that the state comes and does an evaluation because there's been horrible atrocities in the past. I think it's good that we're policed and doing what we're supposed to be doing." But she also confided, "It is incredibly nerve-wracking having somebody over your shoulder looking at everything that you do and combing through with a fine-tooth comb and looking for anything we did wrong. And not anything that you did right because the right stuff doesn't get mentioned; it's only the wrong stuff." The theme that the focus of the state is placed misguidedly on the letter of the law as expressed through documentation rather than on the more global questions of whether or not residents are happy with their care, not to mention whether the facility is adequately staffed, caused the managers to feel as if their "real" work—emotional and social care of residents—was invisible. Dawn, the manager of the subacute unit at Rolling Hills, explained, "You know you can do everything geared for that patient that's right but if the regulations say it's not, it doesn't matter." She added, "That is a very frustrating part of this job." Heather, Dawn's counterpart at Golden Bay put it another way: "You know [state inspectors] will always find things. And you're made to feel like such a failure. And you know I think we do really well here. There are a lot of great people, caring people here." This summed up the attitudes of the managers who were closely involved in the survey process. They felt that the state was overly focused on the mechanics of documentation and did not understand or appreciate the true nature of the work that they do. "Staff do so much, that people have no idea what they do," Heather explained.

In addition, the daily round of reminders from the administrators and directors of nursing to say certain things or not say certain things to the inspectors enhanced the pressure. Joanne and Lucy, the directors of nursing, routinely used the daily managers meetings as an opportunity to tell staff how to act during the inspection. At one of those meetings Joanne announced that she was continuing to prepare for the inspection (she did not know at the time it would not begin for another two months), and then she coached all in the room what to say if an inspector asked them the procedure for suspected resident abuse. Joanne told them the first priority is always to protect the resident, and only after the resident is safe from harm should the alleged abuse be reported immediately. Then Joanne told the managers to tell the nursing assistants the same thing, because the surveyors would almost certainly ask some of them exactly this question. Andy agreed and added, "That's a feeler for them," meaning that if staff cannot answer that question correctly it will lead the inspectors to ask more probing questions. Andy said that when the state finds a violation, no matter how trivial, the inspectors "keep digging into it." To prepare for the potential digging, corporate supervisors carried out mock surveys and conducted random audits of medical charts, much like they conducted mock audits of Medicaid reimbursement documentation.

Jamie, the only full-time and licensed social worker for more than one hundred residents at Rolling Hills, similarly reminded her colleagues what to expect when the inspection began. She referenced the Nursing Home Reform Act of 1987 to explain how the documentation for state inspections interfered with her ability to spend time with residents and their families. She told a story about how not long after the passage of the law an inspector said he was required to cite the facility for inadequate social services even though it was clear, based on his observations and interviews, that she was doing a good job. The problem, he told her, was that she had not documented that quarterly care plan meetings had occurred. This was a cautionary tale she told to staff: "Because we hadn't taken the time to document it, theoretically we hadn't done it." Jamie described the state inspectors as uncompromising technocrats with a single-minded focus on regulatory compliance, at the expense of more important aspects of care.

Stacey, the wound care nurse at Golden Bay, used a familiar metaphor to describe the preparation for the inspection. She said it is like hosting a dinner party. Before your guests arrive, she explained, you clean up the house and make it look really nice. The guests know that the house is not usually so clean and well kept, but everyone plays along with the pretense that the house always looks that way. To extend the metaphor, much of Stacey's housecleaning entailed catching up on documentation. As the wound care specialist, she was responsible for managing wounds caused by pressure ulcers, which can be lethal if not treated adequately. Yet Stacey said, "I consider the documentation to be my job. I really do see myself as the thing that stands between us and a lawsuit." About the survey, she declared, "Everything has to be completely up to the moment. All my charting has to be done week to week and the reality of it is that sometimes I'm a whole month behind. I have the information but actually going to the chart and putting it in there is a different story." There is a lot of redundant documentation, and it does get in the way of direct care, but the written records about wound management really are important for diagnosis, treatment, follow-up, and of course any potential legal proceedings in which care of pressure ulcers could be implicated. Stacey's preparation is itself part of the system of regulatory compliance.[7]

"The Show"

The managers at both nursing homes were preoccupied for months with the looming inspections. The floor staff, however, had a very different experience than the managers. Floor staff were often unaware of pending inspections by CMS and they explained that they just went about their work as usual. They did, however, notice the managers' behavior change as the inspection approached, and from their perspective it looked like managers were putting on a "show" for the state.

Take Doris, for example. Doris was a nursing assistant at Golden Bay, but she had a much more important position than her job title implies. She helped nursing assistants who needed an extra pair of hands, but she primarily served as a unit clerk, organizing rehabilitation appointments, welcoming visitors, calling 911 when necessary, and processing new admissions and discharges for the busiest unit at Golden Bay—the subacute rehabilitation unit. She also was a crucial link between floor staff and managers and informally represented "the voice of the CNAs" to the managers at Golden Bay. During their inspection, I bumped into her in the hallway and asked how it was going. She chuckled and then suggested I go upstairs to the unit and take a look, "and you can tell me what you think!" We rode the elevator up one floor to the unit, which was unusually quiet, clean, and orderly. On this unit there was typically quite a bit of ambient noise around the nursing station coming from various machines and conversations. It rarely sounded like a therapeutic environment, but it did during the inspection. No lunch carts sat in the hallway, no one was chatting behind the nursing station, and the television was set at a very low volume. Doris made eye contact with me and asked in a tone slightly above a whisper, "What do *you* think?" I thought it looked like they had cleaned up before a dinner party. Down the hallway I saw Carissa, the nurse mentioned in the previous chapter who challenged Crystal over documentation. I figured her day was busy and it was, but not for the reasons I expected. Her busy day, she said, included a new admission as well as a discharge to coordinate, in addition to her everyday duties like distributing medications throughout the day to twenty residents. In other words it was a "routine" busy day, not busy because of the CMS inspectors in the building. She explained to me that the inspectors did not really change her daily work unless they asked her a question, and then she answered to the best of her knowledge. She did find it notable though that Lucy, the director of nursing, arrived at six thirty that morning and personally cleaned the public areas of the unit.

During the inspections, managers hurried around the nursing home while floor staff seemed to work on their routine tasks at a normal pace. While the managers experienced stress and anxiety and seemed to have more tasks to do than they could accomplish in a day, the nursing assistants said that their daily work was easier during the inspections because it was the only time that managers helped them pass out lunch trays, pour water for residents, and assist in other routine CNA tasks. Daphne, a nursing assistant, put it bluntly, "It's a show for the inspectors." She explained that it was the only time managers helped. Ironically, she said, "I wish they would do surprise inspections so they could see what it's really like here!" Daphne did not know the inspections are unannounced. This indicates the remarkable degree to which nursing homes are organized as steep top-down operations. Nursing assistants had basically no participation in meetings to discuss or prepare for the inspections, but watched as managers showed up on the unit to assist in daily care during the inspection. Given that perspective, it rather easily appeared that the managers knew when the survey would begin.

When I asked Bonnie, a nursing assistant at Rolling Hills, about the survey, she rolled her eyes and said, "Oh yeah, we put on quite a performance for [the Department of Public Health]. We do. We can pull anything together when they're here." When asked how her daily work changes during the survey, she responded, "Do I do anything differently? No, I just have to do less of it because we have all this extra help." Marlene concurred: "That's about the only time you see people down there helping other people. I mean this woman that comes in to do the state surveys cannot be that stupid. You see people from the woodwork come down to pass trays, and the first thing they do is [ask a nursing assistant] 'who's this person' [resident]? Well, geez, it's kind of obvious that you don't do it very often." She restated for emphasis, "It just makes me wonder what these people are thinking from the state who come in, and they must see it at every nursing home."

These nursing assistants made an important point. During the inspections at both nursing homes, the managers passed out lunch trays and assisted with other tasks that are normally done by nursing assistants. With unit staffing of about four nursing assistants and two nurses for forty residents who have different dietary needs and require varying levels of assistance, it takes quite some time to pass out all the trays, particularly given the considerable likelihood that a nursing assistant may be tied up helping a resident in the bathroom during mealtime. Chronic understaffing is quite apparent during meal times and other moments of care work that occur in groups rather than as dyads. I think the managers also thought that when they helped to pass trays or make beds it made the nursing home appear to be a more "caring" place, but that was secondary to the desire of nursing homes to be seen providing care that was within regulatory code. In nursing home care, a "fully staffed" shift is still an understaffed shift.[8] The state inspectors were not naïve enough to believe that managers spent their mornings doing work typically done by nursing assistants. The inspectors played along. For example, they did not ask the nursing assistants if managers typically helped with the direct care work, nor did the nursing assistants make clear that this help was provided only when CMS was in the building. Chronic understaffing has been normalized not only by nursing homes but also by the agencies that monitor nursing homes.

Rolling Hills

I walked toward the entrance to Rolling Hills on what had been, so far, a fairly typical morning. It was around eight fifteen, early enough to help with the end of breakfast service before attending the daily managers meeting. I planned to spend time after the meeting helping with activities on the dementia unit, and then I was going to assist the nursing assistants by handing out lunch to residents. But as I approached, I noticed that there was a document taped to the large, white front door. It was a public notification that the Department of Public Health was currently conducting an inspection, and that they were available to speak with visitors. Unsure if Andy or Joanne would ask me to leave, I opened the door cautiously and walked quietly down the hall and into the activities office. Liz, the activities manager, walked out from behind her desk and greeted me enthusiastically: "It's show time!" Her tone was reminiscent of vaudeville or a circus ringleader. She explained, "They haven't gotten to the floors yet, that's when the real dog and pony show will begin" while she pantomimed juggling with her hands.

I was eager to observe the inspection, but was not sure that Andy or Joanne would allow it. I also worried that I might, for some reason, get the facility in trouble. Out of an abundance of caution, I did not want to have to explain my project to the state, even though I had obtained ethics board approval for the study months earlier. I also felt that if inspectors began to ask questions of me or about me, my project could become a distraction to the nursing home. During the survey I wore my company-issued name tag prominently, stuck closely to staff members, and tried to blend in as a volunteer activities assistant, which I was in some respects.

I walked with Nancy, the staff educator at Rolling Hills, as she hastily went through the units to give the floor staff what she called a "refresher" about some of the basic rules of care. Nancy was tall and wiry, with curly red hair and a matter-of-fact tone of voice. She moved quickly to get to the staff before the inspectors did. She pressed the key code to open the lock on the dementia unit's doors, and we walked inside together. She approached Stephanie and Caryn, two LPNs, at the nursing station. Nancy promptly informed them that the state was here for their inspection and asked them to recite the differences among universal, contact, and standard precautions. Nancy's brusque tone had Stephanie so flustered that she broke out in hives. They answered sufficiently, and Nancy turned and marched down the hallway. She asked a housekeeper what to do if she suspected resident abuse. The housekeeper responded correctly that the first thing to do was make sure the resident was safe. Then she left the unit and went into the kitchen, the source of previous inspection violations, and directed the dietary staff how to interact toward the inspectors. "Don't freeze up, don't try and snow them, just answer to the best of your ability." She told them something I heard more than occasionally in the preparation for the survey, "If an inspector asks you something that you're not sure of" she said, "say that you don't know and that you will check and get back to them." Then she reminded them, "No gloves in the dining room, wash your hands good, everyone wear name tags, even if it's just a strip of tape with your name on it." Nancy typically spent very little time in the kitchen, so perhaps she did not know that the dietary staff did all of that already.

The inspection continued at Rolling Hills for three days. I was surprised at how much of the survey was based on observations. Although inspectors spent a lot of time reading charts, they did so from behind nursing stations during the busy day shift. This afforded them the opportunity to observe a number of routine tasks such as the medication pass to residents, meal service, and answering resident call bells. At times they stood next to staff and observed them perform direct care. The inspectors also had the opportunity to speak with residents. At Rolling Hills, the inspectors interviewed a group of higher-functioning residents who served on the "Resident Council," a nominal governing body with no real power that represented the residents' collective voice.[9] Liz was nervous because this was one moment during the inspection when the facility was less able to manage the impressions given off to the state. Nobody knew what the residents would say. Liz stood anxiously outside the door to the room where the meeting took place, trying to listen in and occasionally looking through the door window. She was concerned that someone might speak negatively or inaccurately about the facility, but was hopeful that the residents were in a good mood because many of them had recently received free manicures from volunteer cosmetology students.[10] Meanwhile, managers hurried past us, up and down the hallway. The facility was never more clean, quiet, and orderly, and the floor staff enjoyed more help from the managers than at any other time in my observations.

Golden Bay

The managers at Golden Bay had waited months for the inspectors. Finally, at the very end of the six-month survey window, the inspectors arrived on a blustery autumn morning. Crystal called to alert me that they were on site, and when I arrived a few hours later I saw the familiar note on the front door that indicated the inspection was under way. I walked in quietly and saw Cynthia dart down the hallway and into her office. No sooner than I set my bag down in the financial office did Lucy open the door and tell Crystal and her office mate Dorothea, "I need you on the units." Lucy closed the door and Crystal griped that she had work to do, and wondered aloud, "How must it look to the state when we have managers barreling up and down the unit?" Lucy, the director of nursing, had a plan. She directed managers who were not typically on the units to monitor various stations throughout the nursing home. Crystal complained to me that the tactic was transparent: "We're putting on a show and everyone knows it." She thought it was too obvious, but she was also opposed on the grounds that managers such as herself who have "money positions" should continue to do their work because of its critical importance to the facility. Besides, she said, it was obviously unusual for managers to be milling around on the units.

Crystal went reluctantly to her station on the dementia unit, and I walked around to take in the scene. I caught up with Patricia, the staff educator, who praised the idea of the inspections but also said it was nerve-wracking, in the main hallway. I walked with her as I did with Nancy during Rolling Hills' survey, and watched as she did a range of tasks that she virtually never did any other time. She tidied up common areas, monitored hallways, served lunch to residents, and generally walked around and cleaned whatever needed it. She also pulled members of the floor staff aside and asked them to sign documents necessary for their employee file to be completely up to date. Dorothea was stationed on the long-term care unit all day. Susan, the lead social worker, monitored the rehabilitation unit while Lucy and Cynthia walked up and down the halls constantly and tucked into their offices to confer on and off throughout the day.

Dave, the maintenance director, and I did not speak to each other much, but during the inspection we found ourselves walking toward each other from opposite ends of the main hallway. As I passed him, he told me, "This is a good time to observe. This is the way it's supposed to be every day." I took his cue, stopped, and replied, "You mean, quiet and orderly?" He chuckled and said, "Yeah, exactly." The next morning, he had good news to report. He said that an inspector told him that the facility looked so good that they did not even require an inspection. Lucy reinforced Dave's report because she said a surveyor told her that the facility should be graded on a different scale than its peers because Golden Bay accepted sicker residents than other nursing homes. Privately, Crystal snickered, "I don't believe it. [The inspectors] are just scratching the surface."

About an hour later, Dave approached me as I served snacks and hung out with a few residents. A bigger guy, he leaned in, got close to my ear and whispered, "I need you to do me a favor." Eager to gain his trust, I said "okay" and then asked what he needed. The inspectors sought proof that the holiday garland hanging in the doorways was fire retardant, and Dave had not saved the boxes or any documentation that came with it. He asked me to go to the store and buy a box of the garland, which was clearly labeled flame retardant. He handed me a twenty-dollar bill, and I raced out to the store. After some searching, I found what he wanted. I bought the garland and saw Dave as I walked into the facility. He was in the main dining room. From a distance I discreetly held up the plastic bag and nodded, and he gave me a "thumbs-up" and pointed me into the financial office. Moments later he came in, looked in the bag, ripped the label off the box, and quickly left to show the surveyor. He came back ten minutes later, obviously successful, and told me "great job." So even I got into the act.[11]

As the survey wound down, I noticed that the managers' collective mood began to change. It became clear that there were some problems. At the morning meeting, Cynthia said the surveyors were preparing to leave but cautioned her staff to "watch what you say." Then she chuckled pensively and said with a cross between a smile and a grimace, "No one say it's been months since a resident has had glasses on!" Apparently an inspector noticed that a resident on the dementia unit who was supposed to be wearing glasses was not wearing them. He asked the nursing assistant where the glasses were, and she told him that the resident had not worn glasses for months. It seemed as if the resident's glasses got lost and nobody noticed or took action to get her a new pair.

Cynthia also privately told me she was disappointed at how the inspectors had interpreted the circumstances around a resident fall. She was worried it would result in a "G-level" citation. Behind the nursing station of the reha-bilitation unit, she told me about a resident who fell in the dayroom when her family was visiting. The state was going to cite the facility, she feared, because there were no staff in the room assisting or watching the resident. Cynthia explained that they were trying to give the resident some privacy with her family and it would have been inappropriate for a staff member to be there. Instead, the inspectors suggested that the nursing home staff should have been there given the plan of care for that resident. Cynthia lamented that the state was so preoccupied with placing blame that they lost sight that some falls were simply not preventable. The managers were worried about this fall in particular because it resulted in a fracture, and if the facility was found culpable, it would be the second consecutive survey that they would be cited for "falls with fractures," a violation for which the penalty could be quite severe.

Encore, Encore

Months of preparations for several days of intense performance turned into a set of claims made by the state about the quality of the nursing homes. Andy and Joanne were hired precisely because of their strong records with inspections, something that had historically plagued Rolling Hills. Prior to their arrival, the Department of Public Health "blasted this building." Andy said, "That's why they hired me." Andy had previously taken the helm at nursing homes with poor inspection records and improved them. Andy was optimistic after the inspectors left, describing their efforts as "fantastic" and "rock solid." He praised the staff and credited Joanne for her preparation, but also for her reputation. That was the reason why the inspectors were "giving us the benefit of the doubt now" whenever there was a problem that bordered on a deficiency and inspectors had authority to use discretion. Andy did have a lingering concern that the circumstances that led to a resi-dent's fall would result in a damaging "G-level" deficiency. He and Joanne argued that the fall merited a less severe "D-level" care plan deficiency rather than a "G-level" citation that found the nursing home responsible for doing harm to a resident.

The official results arrived by mail several weeks after the survey. Exhibit-ing some confidence and transparency, Andy opened the large, flat envelope in front of the managers. Andy was elated to find that there were only a few deficiencies and zero "G-level" citations. The fall was found to be the result of a "D-level" deficiency. They also got a "D-level" tag for improper handling of resident grievances. They also were cited for low food temperatures. Andy told the group that "this is a very, very good survey," and he was pleased to find "no surprises." But the survey process was not over. Nursing homes are required to respond to all deficiencies with a plan of correction that must be approved by the state inspectors after it is implemented. For instance, their plan to correct low food temperatures included random testing of the food temperatures and timing how long it took to deliver food to residents after it left the kitchen. These were fairly routine diagnostics, and the managers were relieved and proud that they had done so well, particularly compared to how the facility had done before Andy and Joanne took over. It underscored their feeling that the facility was headed in the right direction.

At Golden Bay, the anxiety that crept into the managers' conscious-ness toward the end of the inspection was well founded. When the survey results came back they had around ten violations. This was not good by any standard. Some of them were "G-level" deficiencies, both related to falls that had resulted in fractures. They also had a violation for not keep-ing the physical environment "free of dangers that cause accidents." That meant that a lunch cart or some other piece of equipment was found left in the hallway during the inspection. A few other violations reflected what managers believed to be poor documentation rather than poor care. For example, after the survey results came in, Crystal said, "Someone needs to teach the nurses how to write." And when I asked what she meant, her col-league Dorothea called it "cover-your-ass writing." They described a way to document that does not implicate yourself or the facility that is not taught in the formal curriculum of nursing school, but savvy nurses know how to do it. Crystal and Dorothea, as managers and long-time nurses, knew how to write notes in the chart that are accurate without implicating the facility with any potential wrongdoing.

The inspection report was so severe that CMS imposed a daily fine until the nursing home had responded to the state's findings with a comprehen-sive plan of correction. Cynthia told me that Golden Bay was fined more than twenty thousand dollars, and she gave me a copy of the fifty-seven item plan to correct the deficiencies. The state would return in several weeks to certify the implementation of the plan of correction. The plan of correc-tion included a number of measures to identify and care for residents who were at the highest risk of falling down, including the implementation of a weekly, interdisciplinary "falls meeting" in which every fall was assessed for its "root cause," ensuring that staff had proper follow-up from physi-cians after a fall and that the nursing home keep a more thorough record of how well care plans were being followed. For another part of the plan of correction, Lucy determined that more than 50 percent of all residents and about 80 percent of residents on the long-term care unit were at high risk of falling. She created a binder that contained the care plans for the high-fall-risk individuals and ordered all the rehab therapists, about a dozen people, to read them and initial the binder when they went to the units. Kirstan, the rehab coordinator, looked exasperated when Lucy introduced this new paperwork, and she said, "I don't know how I'll get them to do that." It appeared that, even with the deficiencies, she did not think this was a reasonable or helpful request. Lucy said the rationale was that the rehab therapists should know who is unable to walk safely so they can assist and hopefully prevent a fall.

Things at Golden Bay got worse before they got better. After the plan of correction was submitted but before the state had returned to certify it, four residents fell accidentally. I observed a particularly tense "falls meeting" the following week. All four falls were discussed, and Lucy sat at the head of a table with an open binder and took notes meticulously on the discussion. She said they had to do a "root cause analysis" of the falls to find out why they occurred and how to prevent them. When I started fieldwork there, I noticed paper signs underneath the glass-topped conference table that reminded the staff to do a "root cause analysis," although I was not sure what that meant at the time. I asked a manager what they were there for, and she explained they were part of the previous plan of correction, in which they were also cited for resident falls.

About halfway through the meeting, Cynthia walked into the conference room and joined the meeting. She told them, "I know everyone's been feeling down lately, but this will make you feel better," and she curiously glanced at me and motioned my way as she said that. Perhaps she was self-conscious that I was observing a sensitive meeting at a precarious time for the nursing home. Cynthia said that the four falls over the last week would not be held against them for the survey they just had, nor would they count as falls that had occurred since the implementation of the plan of correction. In other words, these falls fell through the cracks of regulatory code: they occurred after the previous survey but before the implementation of the plan of correction. She was saying the facility would not be held accountable to the state for these falls. Debby, the manager of the dementia unit, reacted with righteous indignation: "That's supposed to make me feel better?" she said. "I would feel better if we really had no falls last week, or if I didn't have any residents sent out to the hospital." Debby's comment was uncharacteristically confrontational, as she took the moral high ground over the administrator. The implication was that all Cynthia cared about was the inspection results, whereas Debby was more concerned with the residents.

In the falls meeting, the staff discussed Virginia, a resident who was allowed to walk independently, despite her Parkinson's disease and history of psychotic symptoms. She had fallen recently, not for the first time. The inspectors said Virginia was not competent to make that decision on her own. Some staff members agreed, but others did not. A few said that Virginia would simply do whatever she wanted, regardless of what they decided. As the managers discussed how to proceed, Cynthia stopped the debate cold when she said, "The bottom line is that we can't let anyone fall." If the facility got cited again for the same falls-related deficiencies, it would be three consecutive surveys and the facility would be penalized severely with a citation for "poor quality management." There was some discussion about using restraints on Virginia, a rare occurrence since the implementation of the 1987 Nursing Home Reform Act, which dramatically narrowed the scope of allowable restraint use.[12] Susan said, "If we use restraints then they're going to say we're taking away their rights." Cynthia explained, "We need to protect the facility," and Jim said it seemed like the state wanted them to shift the benefit of the doubt away from Virginia's mental competency and toward her being incompetent to make decisions. The staff decided that Virginia was no longer safe to walk independently. They would install a motion sensor alarm in Virginia's room to alert the staff in case she got up to walk. In addition to the sensor, they would have a staff member accompany Virginia wherever she walked. The survey process did improve the facility's response to falls in an effort to prevent them in the future, and thus the inspection seemed to do exactly what it was intended to do. Yet this remedy, a nursing assistant to walk with a fall-risk resident wherever she went, also took the assistant away from the other nine residents she was to care for, exacerbating the pervasive understaffing and work overload.

The state inspectors returned several weeks later to review the implementation of the plan of correction. Cynthia and Lucy were, as during the initial inspection, walking quickly through the facility to remind staff members of the new procedures established by the plan of correction. For example, Lucy reminded Terry, the activities director, not to forget that the individuals who were deemed to be at high risk of falling had to sit at their own table so they could be more closely monitored. Terry had the table ready, and said that all her staff had signed the documentation to acknowledge the new procedure. The follow-up inspection took a day, and although Cynthia and Lucy were obviously stressed, it went smoothly and a few days later the state notified them that they had approved the plan of correction, ending the survey process for the next nine months until the new survey window opened.

The performative aspects of the inspection ensured that all parties to the performance normalized understaffing and work overload. Goffman wrote that performances may become a source of cohesion in otherwise stratified spaces: "Where staff and line statuses tend to divide an organization, performance teams may tend to integrate the divisions."[13] The inspectors are not gullible; they know a lot about how nursing homes operate. They know that managers, especially the managers who hold money positions, do not typically pass out lunch trays and assist with activities. Yet they accept the legitimacy of the act. The floor staff also maintained the performance. They did not tell the inspectors that managers help with the everyday care work only when the inspectors are present. This is the open secret of the inspection, and it is a secret that allows for the implicit acceptance of chronic understaffing.[14]

Although I used performance metaphors to describe staff behavior, the inspections were more than an act. Much of Goffman's work is premised on the well-known statement by the sociologist W. I. Thomas in 1928: "If men define situations as real, they are real in their consequences." Meaning is constructed, and those meanings we construct shape our behavior. The inspection process reveals a curious inversion of the Thomas theorem. The situation was defined as an unreal performance for the state. Yet all parties involved viewed the consequences of the performance as a deadly serious matter, and they behaved accordingly. A situation defined as unreal—a show—can also be real in its consequences. The key consequence is the normalization of one of the most severe operational challenges in nursing home care—understaffing.

Despite the normalization of understaffing, the inspections imposed a kind of institutional memory about the formal rules of care. Staff should be reminded about these rules every so often, especially given their high turnover rates.[15] The inspection, then, is not the meaningless charade that the language of the stage implies. Quite the contrary; it is precisely because of the survey's material consequences that staff spent so much time and energy preparing for it. Perhaps this is what Goffman implied when he dropped the language of the stage on the penultimate page of *The Presentation of Self in Everyday Life*. "Scaffolds," he wrote, "are to build other things with, and should be erected with an eye to taking them down. This report is not concerned with aspects of theater that creep into everyday life. It is concerned with the structure of social encounters—the structure of those entities in social life that come into being whenever persons enter one another's immediate physical presence."[16] The act that Goffman is concerned with, and that I am concerned with in this chapter, has real consequences. The improvements made in the name of preparing for inspections and correcting deficiencies improve some aspects of care—because of the performance. The nursing homes put on shows. The inspectors see shows. But these shows matter because, to put them on, the nursing homes have to do real things that improve care. However, in legitimizing the performance, inspections may also do harm by normalizing the real long-term consequences of inadequate staffing ratios and work overload found in nursing homes across the country. If inspectors ask questions about why or how often the nurse managers are doing tasks typically reserved for low-wage staff like nursing assistants and maintenance, they will open up the Pandora's box of nursing home care. Staffing problems plague nursing home care and structure the work routines and the emotional strategies of care workers who struggle to provide good care and also to dignify their work. The inspection process focuses on other issues that are certainly relevant and important for care, but doing that elides very important problems that structurally undermine nursing home care work.

One key question this chapter has left unanswered is why the survey results were better at Rolling Hills than at Golden Bay (particularly given the financial trouble Rolling Hills faced, discussed in further detail later in the book). I am not sure the reason *why* is truly knowable, but I can offer three possible explanations. Golden Bay admitted individuals who needed more acute care, and coordinating that care is more difficult and has greater potential for mistakes. As discussed in the previous chapter, residents who need more care also reimburse more, so perhaps the results reported here are part of a pattern connected to reimbursement incentives to take more clinically acute residents. This could also explain why for-profits such as Golden Bay generally have higher deficiencies than do nonprofits, because for-profits could be more likely to take the highest reimbursing residents. Second, Cynthia argued that there is wide variation in deficiency citations depending on who is doing the inspections. As Golden Bay was preparing the plan of correction, she told me that she attended a seminar that presented data showing substantial regional variation within the state and between states that, she argued, undermines the validity of the survey. This could certainly play a role as well, since part of the reason Rolling Hills hired Joanne as director of nursing was because she had a productive relationship with state inspectors and those network ties could have an impact on overall deficiency scores. Much like the Medicaid auditors, state inspectors have considerable discretion as street-level bureaucrats to interpret and apply regulatory standards. The third explanation is simply that the survey results are not a good predictor of nursing home quality. Staff members across the work hierarchies of both nursing homes stated repeatedly that the inspections were not a good measure of nursing home quality, and my findings support that to a certain extent. It is quite possible, and probably quite common, for a nursing home to be in regulatory compliance while also normally understaffed.

3

Documenting Conflict

Nursing home managers are subject to significant constraints and pressures from the financial and regulatory structure to treat care as a sequence of reimbursable acts. In a system that essentially does not provide enough resources, the managers do what they can to squeeze every dollar out of Medicaid without crossing the fraud line, and they maintain regulatory compliance with performative measures that leave systemic understaffing and work overload in place. The managers are themselves subject to these demands in order to keep the nursing homes financially afloat, but they are torn and struggle to reconcile the tensions inherent in this system. Despite real differences in the managerial orientation of the two nursing homes (for-profit/nonprofit), the logic of the reimbursement and regulatory system forced managers in both facilities to orient their practices in basically the same way. Both nursing homes operated within the same structure and were subject to the demands those structures generate.

An extensive scholarly literature compares nursing home outcomes along a wide range of variables.[1] These variables, such as profit status, reflect fundamental differences between nursing homes across the country. In my research, however, I found that the key difference in nursing home care—especially as it pertains to the experience of work—lies not between nursing homes, but within them. Everyone throughout the organizational chain wanted to provide good care, but the meaning of good care differed depending on position within the organizational hierarchy. The floor staff constructed care in zero-sum terms—time spent on documentation was time not spent on caring. Caring involved meeting the physical, emotional, and social needs of residents, and that was the floor staff's priority. Documentation was separate and secondary. From the managers' perspective, documentation was a critical element of good care; not only did it provide a written record the staff could use to develop care plans, it also protected the facility legally.

Previous research looking at nursing home care, such as Diamond's ethnography *Making Gray Gold*, has shown that managers in nursing homes use the mantra of "If it's not documented, it didn't happen" to explain the importance of documentation. I too found that managers used that exact phrase. Cynthia, the administrator at for-profit Golden Bay, put it more mildly, as she occasionally asked, "Are we doing what we are documenting, and are we documenting what we are doing?" Most important for the nursing homes, documentation was the basis for reimbursements and thus the foundation of the financial viability of the workplace. Floor staff and managers used different interpretive frames to make sense of their work, and these interpretive frames were expressed most clearly in their approaches toward the documentation. The documentation pulls the staff together; workers on the floor and at the management levels have to deal with components of the documentation and, in the process, deal with each other. Yet it also pushed them apart. The seemingly innocuous documentation compelled the floor staff and managers to engage with each other's conceptions of care work, which generated habitual conflict throughout the workplace hierarchies. The managers generally thought that the nursing assistants did not care or were not smart enough to document correctly, and went through multiple rounds of trying to teach the nursing assistants about the financial implications of documentation. The floor staff generally thought that the documentation was just about money and that it undermined and in some crucial ways missed the substance of their care work.

Paper Documentation and the CareTracker

While conflicts between the floor staff and managers played out similarly in both nursing homes, they used different documentation systems to chart residents' behavior. The nonprofit Rolling Hills used a traditional pen-and-paper system, while the for-profit Golden Bay used a new electronic kiosk system called the CareTracker. Just before shift change at Rolling Hills, nursing assistants spent the last twenty to thirty minutes of each workday writing the day's documentation. They tended to gather together around a table or behind the nursing station and one by one they opened the documentation folders for each resident and filled out the "CNA Flow Sheet" that codified the level of assistance provided for standard daily activities such as bathing, getting dressed, and so on. The scale used to determine reimbursement rates ranged from "independent" to "limited assist," "extensive assist," and "total assist." Other parts of the flow sheets required nursing assistants to document how many caregivers were needed to provide adequate assistance for activities such as transferring residents between their beds and wheelchairs. The document itself was straightforward; the big problem for the floor staff was the lack of adequate staffing to document and provide care at the same time. Each CNA did the care and documentation for about ten residents every day (plus or minus two depending on staffing and how many residents are on the unit). As alarms rang or call bells flashed, the nursing assistants eyeballed each other to determine whose turn it was to stop writing their documentation and attend to the residents' needs. Angela, a nursing assistant on the rehabilitation unit, described how pressing care needs could derail the documentation:

> When we're doing our charting as a group, and there's all kinds of talking, then you've got lights to answer, and then you've got nursing saying, "Could so-and-so please bring Mr. Papadakis down to the podiatrist?" So, "Okay, I'll get up" and so I went over, got Mr. Papadakis. He was resting in bed, so I told him that the podiatrist was here, wanted to look at his toenails. So I helped him up in the chair and brought him down there to the podiatrist. But then on the way back, instead of going to the charts I stopped in to answer another light and brought that resident to the bathroom and then back. So I'm thinking, "Oh man, if I sit down across from the nurses' station again and have to get back up and answer lights." So I ran, got my charts, and I do need to go to a quiet spot, because in order to chart on ten residents you need a good block of time.

In addition to the constraints of chronic understaffing, there was the mismatch between the flow of care throughout the day and the way the state measures care. Residents' needs vary during each shift in ways that cannot be documented on the Flow Sheet. Stephanie, a nurse who was promoted to management by the time my fieldwork ended, explained it in our interview. She said, "The documentation is confusing. Sometimes people are both incontinent and continent in the same day. You know, money talks, and I've told them guys [management], you know, give a training because the CNAs have to document that they're incontinent, but they're both." As Stephanie pointed out, when residents were continent and incontinent on the same shift, there were two viable choices for only one box. They did this documentation inconsistently because the behaviors they care for are themselves inconsistent. Thus the reimbursement system built around turning care into discrete reimbursable acts generates conflict within nursing homes; as discussed in the chapter on Medicaid reimbursement, the managers push nursing assistants to document residents as the most dependent on staff as possible without crossing the fraud line because it raises reimbursements.

It is not only that documentation cannot adequately capture the character of round-the-clock care work. The larger problem is that each nursing assistant is tasked with, at the very least, maintaining the safety of ten residents, most of them in various stages of memory loss and physical decline. Given this context it is not difficult to understand how documentation could take second priority to direct care work. Take Caryn, for example, a nurse at Rolling Hills who used to be manager but said she preferred floor work to a "desk job." She lamented that the documentation often got in the way of direct care, describing it as "just a lot of redundancy. I mean, we're writing the same thing in ten places sometimes. That's ridiculous. Ridiculous." Alice, a career nursing assistant with more than twenty years of experience, explained, "I personally care more about the residents—I mean than if paperwork gets done. *Hello!* The resident comes first. If the resident's up and acting out, doing whatever, you spend your time with the resident. Paperwork is paperwork, something the state wants. It's ridiculous to me that the state looks at everything that they shouldn't, and overlooks the things that they should." Their accounts were often framed in these terms—caring about documentation was tantamount to not caring about care.

The floor staff tried to resist the push to document for the sake of reimbursement by developing interpretive strategies to account for the motives of management. They made attributions of intent about managers, explaining that they cared only about money and documentation was the way to get the money. Cindy, the top nursing assistant at Rolling Hills according to her supervisor, told me that she became a nursing assistant to take care of old people and did not realize how much of her job would be documentation. She explained that over the years working on the job, her supervisors had taught her about the importance of the documentation, but she still did not see it their way. She explained, "As far as the facility goes, that's probably the first thing that they want done. But you know what; that's not the way it is. To us that's the least problem. If our residents are taken care of, that's all we care about."

Cindy was not the only nursing assistant who saw the managers as overly focused on documentation. When I first met her, Marlene had been a nursing assistant at Rolling Hills for more than five years. She was short and thin, thoughtful and reserved, with long blonde hair that she pulled back tightly into a bun. Most of her time there had been spent doing direct care on the dementia unit, but she also had picked up odd shifts with the laundry department, as an activities assistant, and in the kitchen as a dietary aide. One morning as we sat in the activities office, she told me rather bluntly, "The unit managers and front office people really don't care about the residents. That's what stresses me out. Those residents should come first, not the money and not whatever else they're thinking about. And sometimes you can't always do your documentation that day. You just don't have time, the residents are more important. They need to see that." What was actually a conflict generated by the reimbursement and regulatory structure of nursing home care came off to Marlene and other floor staff as if the managers did not care about residents.

The managers did care, but they practiced it differently than the floor staff. The floor staff said that the managers wanted them to exaggerate in the documentation how much care was provided because that is how "they" made more money. Victoria at Rolling Hills reviewed the Flow Sheets periodically and left notes for the floor staff about how care should be documented. Although most nursing assistants did not know much about the mechanics of the reimbursement system and its relationship to the documentation, they knew enough to understand that, as it was often said to me, "It's all about the money." Daphne, a nursing assistant, opined, "What we do for the residents sometimes isn't right for management. It's all about the money. When we don't document it the way they want they lose money, because however that works, the insurance—they don't get enough credit, so they don't get paid enough or whatever. But you know, that's been a big issue with the aides because we're telling them, 'We're not going to lie. We're not going to lie about what we do for these residents.' If they can do a lot for themselves, we're not going to put that they're dependent. So that was a big issue." Few characterized what managers asked the staff to do as lying, but they repeatedly asked the floor staff to alter documentation after it was written. Daphne continued, "You know, and it got to the point where—you know, they'd leave little sticky notes, 'Well this is the way it should be charted.' So we'd write notes back, 'Well, this is what we do for them, so this is what we're putting.' So we'd get lectured on it. It's always the money, money, money, money."

Daphne's colleague, Maria, had worked at Rolling Hills for over four years. When she saw notes from Victoria to change documentation that did not seem right, she refused. "I'm just—I just tell them, 'Listen. I didn't do that with her today.' So if I didn't do it, I'm not charting it. I'm not charting what I haven't done. I'm not putting my name on anything that I haven't done and actually done it—you know." Bonnie was a veteran of Rolling Hills, having worked there since the facility opened. She complained about the "stupid little notes from someone that doesn't even know these people" to change her documentation. I asked for a recent example and she said, "Oh, it was a resident that they wanted me to put assist for feeding, and I refused because the person, I had to put independent because the person was eating in the hall alone. And you cannot put someone as an assist if they're eating in the hall alone because if that person chokes and they say, 'Well, why wasn't someone assisting them?'" Bonnie, a nursing assistant, relied on a rhetoric of professionalism and job security to deflect pressures to alter documentation, much like the managers discussed in previous chapters who dealt with the same pressures from their supervisors. Bonnie pointed out the legalities of the documentation that could identify her as a responsible party in case there was an accident. She was, in her mind, not willing to jeopardize her job security so the facility could increase its Medicaid reimbursement.

The conflicts over documentation at Rolling Hills were expressed through the pen-and-paper documentation. The managers at Golden Bay had dealt with similar issues, which is why they had recently installed an electronic system called the CareTracker. The CareTracker may have mitigated the types of conflict that the pen-and-paper system generated, but it created other types of conflict. Lucy, the director of nursing, said they purchased the CareTracker system because the pen-and-paper documentation encouraged floor staff to copy unreflectively the previous documentation even if it was incorrect. Mistakes multiplied. Nursing assistants could not clock out of work until their documentation was complete and the system reset if they walked away from the screen before finishing their documentation, providing some good reasons for nursing assistants to assign greater priority to documentation than they had prior to the installation of the CareTracker. Computer kiosks that looked a lot like the stations wait staff at restaurants use to put through orders to the kitchen were located throughout the units. Instead of sitting together around a table to complete the documentation as a group, like at Rolling Hills, the nursing assistants at Golden Bay took turns standing at the stations entering the documentation via touch screen. The system automatically used terms that were more consistent with the language the state uses to measure and reimburse care; thus it likely produces greater overall reimbursements than the pen-and-paper version. Indeed the CareTracker website boasts that "more than 80% of all CareTracker facilities increase Medicare and Medicaid reimbursement after implementing Care-Tracker."[2] A number of floor staff said that they were slow, provided no way to make notations or provide details, and were positioned too high on the wall, causing the staff neck and shoulder pain.

I asked Doris, the Golden Bay nursing assistant who does work consistent with a unit clerk, about the CareTracker compared to the old pen-and-paper system. Doris had won the nursing home's "Employee of the Year" award more than once. The CareTracker, she explained, diminished her ability to chart using her own vocabulary for behavior. She said, "On paper you can always show something differently for behavior-wise exactly. On the kiosk you got certain categories. So no more can you ever place it in your own wordings." She did not like the CareTracker for the same reasons why the management did like it: "You don't have per se your own thoughts anymore. It's—these are the choices. A lot of the behavior categories, they don't cover every single behavior in the ways that we were taught or know how to stop a behavior or whatever. It's like five choices and these are the only choices. So whether it's exactly what the computer's sayin' or not that's what we would have to chart on. So it's takin' away your own thoughts." The choices provided by the CareTracker corresponded very closely with the state and federal forms, which would likely lead to higher reimbursement because there would be fewer mistakes and increased monitoring from managers. The last thing they wanted was floor staff, whom they considered generally to be not very bright, to freelance the documentation. Rather, they had a specific set of terms that they wanted to see on the documentation, and the CareTracker closely matched those terms and limited the ability of the floor staff to document outside those parameters.

Furthermore, Doris suggested that the documentation is one way in which the staff can attribute functional competence to residents, resisting the idea that residents are the mere embodiment of reimbursable activities. She explained, "I don't like documentation and reimbursement because you're takin' a lot away from a resident. If you do—they're tellin' us if you do one item for the resident, say if you—they needed help just doin' something eating-wise. You strip them from being independent to being limited assist. So now they're documented as limited assist instead of givin' 'em that independence and it's all about money and I understand the importance of documentation and money and all that, but it sucks. I don't like it. I don't like it at all." In other words, she was saying that describing residents as more helpless than they really are undermines their perceived agency. Doris connected the documentation to residents' behavior and the tensions that emerge around labeling a resident as dependent upon staff for routine behaviors. It is important for care workers to make attributions of competence and independence wherever possible, in a sense giving or ascribing agency to residents.[3] The overall push by managers to emphasize the dependence of residents weakened their ability to symbolically give residents agency, something that, as I will show in chapter 7, is essential to how they constructed a dignified moral order in the workplace. Embellishing the dependence of floor staff to increase reimbursement money undermined the ability of floor staff to make attributions of agency about residents. It made it more difficult for staff to construct residents as capable of taking care of themselves at all.

The CareTracker also allowed the managers to monitor the documentation more closely and make alterations more easily. Carla, a nurse at Golden Bay, had previously worked at County Nursing Home, a state-owned nursing home that closed long ago. She preferred to work on the long-term care unit because it afforded her the ability to get to know the residents and their families for some length of time. With her breadth of experience, she realized quickly how the managers could use the CareTracker to manipulate the documentation for financial gain. She stated it bluntly, "When we got the kiosks I went right away and I went to, I actually forget what her name is, but she's the one that oversees Crystal. I says, 'I am not changing my summary to go along with what that employee put on the kiosks because that would be lying, and I'm not doing that.' I says, 'I'm not documenting that something happened so that they can get more money when it's not true and it's actually a change in status for a patient.' I says, 'I am not doing that.'" As Carla noted, the managers could (and did) use the CareTracker to alter documentation to suit their own purposes. The revised documentation had to be signed by the nursing assistant who did the initial entry to approve of the change that was made. Crystal typically sought out those individuals long after the care work in question had been provided, making it easy for the floor staff to acquiesce and sign whatever document their supervisor put in front of them.

Managers and the floor staff did not think explicitly about the documentation as a field in which they struggled for control over the workplace, but it was. The floor staff said that the problems were caused by greed and that the managers misunderstood the nature of work in nursing homes. The workers on the floor of the nursing homes were not unaware of the financial considerations—they cared about care and did not see documentation as a part of care. The managers tried repeatedly to convince the floor staff how much the documentation mattered to the facility, but the floor staff were far more concerned with the meeting the immediate needs of residents. What the managers chalked up as stupidity or just being too busy for proper documentation was actually about a conflict rooted in social structure and how structural position shapes experience and interpretation. This becomes clear upon looking at how the managers and floor staff responded to the conflict, with the managers engaged in a seemingly endless loop of educational efforts to teach floor staff about the money riding on the documentation and the floor staff taking quite a different lesson from the proceedings.

"Educating, and Educating, and Educating, and Reeducating"

Nancy, the staff development coordinator at Rolling Hills mentioned in the previous chapter, spent several years working as a floor nurse prior to being promoted to a management position. She identified with how the floor staff approached the documentation, and explained, "I as a staff nurse resented documentation because I always thought patient care's first and don't bother me with your paperwork and there's too much of it and I'm going to do patient care first. And if that doesn't get done, well, too bad." This is indeed a good summary of the views of the floor staff. When she became a manager and learned the legal protections solid documentation affords, she came to a new understanding of its importance. She could tell that the staff resented the documentation from their body language: "I can almost feel it and I don't know if it's just me projecting it because that's how I used to feel, but yeah. Partly yeah, it's like, 'I'm going to do the patient care first' and it's just that they have so much to do. It's almost like humanly impossible to do everything you have to do and when you have the paperwork on top of it, where's the priority?" Her explanation of how becoming a manager changed her point of view about the documentation captures the significance of structural position within an organization.

Managers like Nancy described the documentation as an essential component of good care and came up with a variety of reasons why the nursing assistants seemed to have so much difficulty seeing the connection. They explained that the nursing assistants did not understand how important the documentation was, or they were not smart enough or too lazy, or they empathized to a degree with the nursing assistants, although in a backhanded way, saying nursing assistants had "bad jobs." They talked more than occasionally derisively about the nursing assistants' abilities. The first day I spoke with Crystal, I asked about the kiosks, and she made zombie-like arm motions and a blank facial expression and said, "Oh, you've probably seen them [nursing assistants] standing there, doing it." In our interview many months later, she added, "I mean how many times have you seen them, kind of blurry-eyed, standing in front of the screen, kind of pecking at it, like a woodpecker really quickly?" As I sat with Crystal and other managers in the financial office, Stacey, the wound specialist, said in her typically blunt, unapologetic style that the nursing assistants "don't know what they're doing." Crystal thought an education campaign might help, which Dorothea, another manager, mocked, "Yeah sure, we'll drill a hole into their skull, pour in the education, and then fill the rest up with cement," which made the group laugh raucously.

At Rolling Hills, I observed a meeting in which the managers' increasing dissatisfaction with the quality of the nursing assistants' documentation had reached a crescendo, exemplifying the opposing priorities at play along the work hierarchy. In the daily managers meeting, Carol, the Medicare reimbursement coordinator, held up the documentation completed by a nursing assistant and pointedly stated that it was "absurd and unprofessional." She explained that the information provided by the nursing assistant was inadequate and that she could not use it to complete the federal documentation required for Medicare reimbursement. Dawn, the manager of the rehabilitation unit, which deals the most with residents who are on Medicare, added that the safety checks, completed every two hours, were signed off for a resident who was dead and for two who had already returned home. This was precisely the kind of error that the Department of Public Health looked for during the inspections. Victoria, the Medicaid reimbursement coordinator discussed in chapter 1, piled on, "Nursing summaries haven't been done in three months!" Joanne, the director of nursing, had reached her boiling point. She had a commanding presence and balanced Andy's enthusiastic and occasionally brash style. Joanne was nearly six feet tall and broad-shouldered, and she styled her short dark hair straight back, away from her face, and she had a rare skill for cutting to the central issue in a debate. She declared, "All this nonsense has to stop. We did not go to any special nursing school, how is it that we [managers] can act professionally and they [nursing assistants] can't?" Joanne said that they had a stable staff now and that "we are no longer held hostage to them, and I am done educating, and educating, and educating, and reeducating them on some of these simple tasks." As the managers nodded in agreement, Joanne called for an all-staff "come to Jesus" meeting.

After the meeting ended I walked to the rehabilitation unit and found Cindy, a nursing assistant. The unit manager, Dawn, described Cindy as "my top CNA. She has a way with patients. She really has a way with families. She takes on the lead. She is a very, very strong leader." True to that description, during my first week of fieldwork Cindy introduced herself to me and was curious to know about my project. We got along well and trusted each other.[4] I trailed her for about an hour between breakfast and lunch as she worked nonstop around the unit. She helped residents in the bathroom, served ice water, took weights, made beds, changed sheets, and showered a resident while his son waited. Then it hit her: she looked at me and said, "Oh my god, I'm gonna get reamed out" because she had forgotten to document the two-hour safety checks (what Dawn had complained about in the meeting). Cindy alerted another nursing assistant that Dawn was going to "ream us out" and that person turned toward us, shrugged her shoulders, and said simply, "I'm agency," which meant she worked for a staffing agency and would perhaps never return to Rolling Hills. Therefore implying that she had nothing to be worried about, she rather coldly turned and walked away. Cindy turned the corner and headed toward the nursing station, and there was Dawn, with the safety check documents in her hand, giving Cindy the stink eye. Cindy explained she was so busy that she did the safety checks but forgot to write them down. Dawn replied that she realized Cindy was busy but needed to remember. Dawn turned toward me, held up the forms, and called out, "See! The documentation!" underscoring the severity of the problem discussed in the meeting I observed. Then she sidled up to Cindy, showed her the documentation, and said calmly, "See this woman? She's in heaven. See these two? They don't live here anymore." She waved the paperwork at Cindy and said, "This is fraud. To the inspectors, this is fraud."

This example highlights and clarifies the tension around documentation between the floor staff and the management. Cindy was working on residents; what I saw when I trailed her was not an unusual day. This was her midmorning routine. It seemed obvious to her that serving water and making beds was more important than initialing documentation. A few months later I interviewed Cindy over lunch. She told me that it is so busy on the unit "and I'll be honest with you, a lot of times we'll go, 'Oh my God, did we do a safety check?' But the thing of it is I know that my residents, when my little Jeanie gets up I make sure she's alarmed.[5] It's not that we're not doing, we're not checking our people; it's just that we're not getting to the paperwork."

I asked Joanne if I could observe the all-staff "come to Jesus" meeting that occurred a week later, but she said no. At the time, she stated her concern that I "might have ulterior motives," but months later she revised her reasoning, explaining that she "was afraid the staff was going to rip me a new one." She did not want me to watch the floor staff embarrass her. Yet I was still able to learn about what transpired at the meeting. I asked members of the floor staff and some managers what occurred. What they told me revealed wildly different interpretations of the point of the meeting.

The managers approached the meeting as an opportunity to educate the floor staff about the critical relationship between documentation and the financial viability of the facility. Everyone gathered in the main dining room for the meeting, which began at three thirty in the afternoon to maximize participation of staff from all shifts. It stretched on for well over an hour.

Carol and Victoria showed the floor staff real examples of incorrect documentation, then what the documentation should have been, followed by the amount of money those mistakes cost the facility. Victoria explained, "I have shown them exactly how much money could be riding on documentation. I've shown them a comparison. I've written out a correct one as opposed to a wrong one, and shown them exactly, you know, right down to the penny how much could be at stake."

Bonnie, a nursing assistant at Rolling Hills for nearly twenty years, was not impressed. She told me, "Honestly, I'm like I could care less what it costs. I mean yes, I do my documentation to the best of my ability, but we're here to take care of the residents, the dollar doesn't matter to me. They're the ones that have to worry about that and are concerned about meeting that almighty budget, not me." At the meeting, "They had done a, I don't know what you'd call it, kind of like an audit type thing and they did it by units to find out the documentation and stuff. And basically what they were trying to prove was that people weren't documenting properly, so we weren't being reimbursed properly, and they were trying to let us know how much money it cost us so that hopefully people would be better about documentation." Yet the meaning she took from the demonstration was not what management had intended, "but it worked in our favor because our unit [dementia unit] had proven through charting that we needed help more than the other floors because of the amount of care and stuff that we were documenting. So our floor was listed as the most difficult, so for a while we got the staffing. And if someone had to be short it wasn't us because we had all this documentation backing us up." To Bonnie, the meeting proved that the dementia unit needed the most staff because their residents needed the most care. Cindy put it differently but also noted how staffing was implicated in poor documentation. She said, "You know, we're taking care of the real things, the hands-on, and it doesn't stop from the time you're there 'til the time you go home. And they're concerned about documentation. And if they're so concerned about it, they need to make a space, a timeframe where you can go and do that. We don't have that. We are hands-on twenty-four seven."

This episode captured the different interpretive frames that the floor staff and managers brought to their understanding of the documentation. For Bonnie and other members of the floor staff, the meeting was a lesson that reinforced the understaffing and work overload they endured as they struggled to do meaningful care work. For Joanne and other members of the management, it was a lesson that reinforced the necessity to document correctly all the care that was reimbursable as they struggled to negotiate a system that reduced nursing home care to a linear stream of instrumental and measurable acts.

At times, managers attributed to the documentation a range of problems centered on the nursing assistants' abilities: they implied that nursing assistants were stupid, lazy, or just did not care. As much as managers blamed the nursing assistants' abilities, some also understood the impact of inadequate staffing resources on the sheer amount of work nursing assistants have to do. Dawn, a unit manager at Rolling Hills, explained, "You know—in their defense, they're busy. CNAs are busy out there. They've got a crappy job." Even Victoria, who said it was "extremely frustrating" to see the same mistakes repeated after she had educated the nursing assistants about the money lost due to incorrect documentation, was sympathetic: "When they're on the floor, and they're doing the hands-on care, it—those patients are the ones in their face, not me [laughs]. So, you know, in their defense, you know, I can— I've been on their end of the deal, too. So I mean; it's a hard job." Carol, the Medicare reimbursement coordinator at Rolling Hills, also saw the problem as partially one of education and partially time constraints. She said, "I think in this facility it's not getting done because their priority is to take care of the patients and documentation comes secondary. But the rules say if you don't document it, you didn't do it, so it's a twofold thing. Everybody's first priority is the patients, but then if you don't go back and document what you did, we can't get credit for it. So that's where the problem lies." Carol is exactly right, but failed to recognize that the tensions she identified are embedded in positions of structural conflict. She explained that nursing assistants become so accustomed to the daily work that they routinely failed to document reimbursable care. This is a big problem to the managers because, as discussed in chapter 1, revenue is lost when reimbursable activities are not documented. She argued, "When you have somebody that's demented and they have these behaviors, whether it's combative, agitation, restlessness, whatever, it's their norm and people just look at it as their norm. Even though you and I wouldn't look at it as being normal behavior, that's where we lack in the documentation because we become so accustomed to each and every individual's idiosyncrasies that we don't see it as abnormal." The nursing assistants, she said, left a lot of reimbursement money on the floors, documenting incorrectly or not at all.

At Golden Bay, when Lucy began as the director of nursing she led a series of trainings about proper documentation. Eventually they faded away, as these things tend to do. Toward the end of my fieldwork, after the annual health and safety inspection revealed serious deficiencies, Lucy organized a series of meetings about documentation. She knew the nursing assistants did not care much about the nursing home finances in the abstract, so she tried to convince them that they had a personal financial stake in thorough documentation of care provided. She explained, "I can say 'if you don't document, we don't get reimbursed.' That doesn't mean a thing to them. You have to put it in terms they can relate to. It's a matter of—can the company afford to give you a 2 percent raise this year or can they give you a 4 percent raise this year?" The documentation is related to the nursing assistant wages abstractly, but there was no explicit connection between the two, especially considering that Golden Bay had recently won awards for their high profitability that did not come with concomitant pay raises for the floor staff.

Lucy's tone was similar to that of her counterpart at Rolling Hills. She said, "If you don't document for the Medicaid, then when Crystal goes to do her MMQ reimbursement with the state, we could lose—if you lose thirty dollars a day times thirty days for six months, you figure it out [$5,400]. And that's only one resident. That money is money *not* in this building, to buy equipment, wages, to replace furniture, or whatever." While reimbursable acts of care that went undocumented was one problem for the managers, Lucy added that the cost of the materials and equipment used in care work also was not recouped because of incomplete documentation. Lucy called out the floor staff,

> When a nurse does a dressing, say they use gauze pads, they're supposed to put it on the charge slip that goes in front of the treatment book. Or if they use D&D Ointment, or do an Accu-Chek for diabetes. You're supposed to write it on the sheet. And at the end of the month it goes to the business office and they charge private insurance, Medicare, or private pay for what is done. If the CNAs and nurses don't charge those things, the building pays for it. So we are paying out thousands and thousands of dollars a month for equipment in this building that could be being charged to insurance companies. So we end up paying for it.

Trying to convince the floor staff that they should care about documentation because the financial health of the nursing home depended on it fell on deaf ears. The floor staff constructed themselves as caring only about the social, emotional, and physical care of residents and to delve into the financial implications of their care undermined those self-conceptions. These different orientations to care were rooted in the hierarchical character of the workplaces. Managers and floor staff worked in different social worlds, with clashing priorities and definitions of care.[6]

Care Plans

The construction and implementation of care plans also reflect the separate orientations of floor staff and managers. Care plans provide a detailed set of step-by-step practices, like a recipe, that list what staff at the point of care need to do to reduce the risk of health complications, such as skin breakdown or falls, that residents may be susceptible to based on the flow sheets and nursing summary documentation. Care plans were written and reviewed every three months, in conjunction with an interdisciplinary care plan meeting that included the manager of the unit that resident lived on, the reimbursement coordinator, a social worker, and the activities coordinator. Sometimes the director of nursing attended. Care practices as they occur on the nursing home floor are ideally entirely consistent with care plans that emerge from the meeting. Lucy, Golden Bay's director of nursing, took pride in her knowledge of the residents. She boasted, "I know all the residents in our building. I could tell you the care plans of just about all of them. And that's not something that most directors of nursing do." That may be true, but care plans reflect a different form of knowledge than the nursing assistant's experiential knowledge, and nursing assistants did not participate in the care plan development.

Occasionally the managers turned explicitly cynical toward the documentation and sounded a lot like the floor staff, suggesting that the care plans were written for the edification of the state. As I observed during a care plan meeting that neither the resident nor the family attended— a common occurrence—the managers in the room were talking to each other and spontaneously began to address their comments to me. Dawn, the unit manager, Jamie, the lead social worker, and Liz, the activities director, were in the room. Jamie said that the documentation took a lot of time away from the residents, and that prior to the 1987 Nursing Home Reform Act she was able to spend more time with residents. Liz lamented, "It's all about money." Dawn, who was often quiet around me, broke her silence and blurted out, "You've been here for a while now, and you see that these residents get good care. They are clean; they are active; they are happy; they eat well." And Jamie in the background said quietly, "There is no odor." Dawn went on, explaining that "none of that matters to the state. They scrutinize the paperwork and if there is any little problem they blow it up into a huge thing, and miss the overall point, which is that the residents are treated well."

Despite these occasional forays into the interpretive frames of the floor staff, that care trumped documentation of care, toward the floor staff they maintained that the care plans were of paramount importance and must be followed on all occasions. Victoria spoke about the care plans in our interview. She explained,

> VICTORIA: The CNAs really need to be in tune to what the care plan says, because if they're doing something not up to what the care plan says, then that can cause its own problems. If the care plan says, you know, this person's a two-assist for ambulation, they're charting one assist, well, there's an inconsistency there.
>
> JASON: Right. So what will happen?
>
> VICTORIA: I'll—you know, I would be the one to say okay, the care plan says this, but you're charting that. What's the discrepancy? This is why I think it should be this way.
>
> JASON: Right.
>
> VICTORIA: And correct it now. [laughs] You know, sometimes the CNAs do have a different view on things, but most of the time the care plans are created from a lot of different assessments, not just one person. I mean, most of the time. You know, they're interdisciplinary care plans, and the interventions are there for a reason. So you know, you've got to go by the care plan.

The managers, like Victoria noted, said that the floor staff had to work according to the care plan directives. The nursing assistants, however, noted that care plans often were inaccurate to their experience with residents. For example, Daphne, who was a nursing assistant in the dementia unit at Rolling Hills for over six years before she left for a position at a nearby hospital, explained, "Well, you know, there were times when, 'cause we're supposed to carry them on us, there were times when I would flip through them and there would actually be residents' names in there who have already passed away, or their statuses have changed and it wasn't changed in their care plans. Or things would be changed and I didn't even know about it, and those are things that should be communicated to me."

Caroline, a newly certified nursing assistant, described the relationship among the documentation, care plans, and the provision of care this way:

> That's confusing because it's supposed to match their care plan, but it's also supposed to match what you do, which doesn't always match the care plan so it's really confusing. If someone's sick, they need more assistance than they normally do and so you have to explain it on paperwork and it's really confusing because you have like nine or ten residents, remembering who

pooped for example and like what size it was, whether it was loose. Out of ten people, you're like okay, who—I don't even remember and then you've gotta remember who washed up and who refused what activities and it's kind of hard to remember.

While nursing assistants at Rolling Hills were supposed to carry the care plans with them, at Golden Bay they were held in a sleeve behind the bathroom door. Nobody looked at them. Crystal and Dorothea, who were the main authors of the care plans, told their colleagues in the daily managers meeting that they spent too much time writing care plans that were ignored by nursing assistants. Cynthia asked Patricia, the staff development manager, to require everyone to read all the care plans and sign a document that certified they had done so. This was a huge request that made Crystal and Dorothea, among others, roll their eyes because they sensed it was unrealistic and felt like it would not happen. To my knowledge it did not.

Despite the apparent mismatch between what the care plans said and the care nursing assistants provided, the consequences for not following the care plan could be severe—for residents and for staff. At one point during my fieldwork at Rolling Hills, Diane, a thirty-year veteran nursing assistant, left a resident alone on the toilet while she passed on information to the oncoming shift, and the resident fell off the toilet and fractured her hip. Hip fractures among the elderly are extremely dangerous; approximately one-quarter of individuals who break a hip die within one year of their injury.[7] Days after the accident, I sat on the floor in the conference room while Joanne, Andy, and the unit manager discussed what to do. They felt badly firing Diane, but Joanne explained, "This building has been repeatedly, and repeatedly, cited for not following the plan of care. Like I said yesterday, you could speed up and down the highway one thousand times, and all it takes is getting caught once. And that's what happened here. Those CNAs think they know the residents. They've been caring for them for years, and they think they know them better than we do, so they don't necessarily follow the plan of care. All it takes is once to see that this is not just an exercise in paperwork." The management fired Diane as a show of force, to prove that care plans matter and that managers knew more about proper care than the nursing assistants. But the managers did not take into account that the nursing assistants could not always follow the care plan because of the time and resource constraints that came from understaffing. It was not that the nursing assistants did not understand the care that residents needed, it was that they were not provided with the resources needed to take care of the residents to the level written in the care plans.

Diane's firing certainly got the attention of the floor staff, but not in the way managers had intended. Rather than increase adherence to the care plan, most of the floor staff viewed Diane's dismissal as unnecessarily harsh. It heightened their sense that the management did not understand the day-to-day work on the floor. A few of the floor staff supported the termination, but most I spoke to opposed it, they said, because Diane was a skilled care-giver who cared about residents. They noted that Diane bought a television for the residents on the dementia unit after the old one broke. They also said she had terrific rapport with residents. Because she had invested so many years at Rolling Hills, it seemed unjust to fire her. Cindy, a respected leader among the floor staff on the rehabilitation unit, was candid: "That's bullshit." Cindy said Diane was a "damn good aide, and she gave them her sweat and her time" and defended her through self-incrimination: "You know, I've left her alone in the toilet myself before to go get a pad and make her bed. You can't—the thing that this facility, they need to know, we have so many tabbed residents there is no, no fucking way that you can stay with one person to be toileted. You will never get your work done."[8] Cindy pointed out that inadequate staffing and meager resources in nursing homes require them to take calculated risks about resident care. The nursing assistants understood the pressures of work overload and judged what Diane had done through a structural lens of being chronically understaffed, while the managers made attributions about Diane as an individual, suggesting that she knew the rules and did not follow them when she could have and should have.

There are several reasons why the implementation and enforcement of the care plans generated such conflict. The first is that the nursing assistants, staff members at the point of care, were systemically excluded from the care plan development process. Serving as the eyes and ears of the homes, nurs-ing assistants were often attuned to small changes in behavior that could reflect the need to change the plan of care. They had something to contribute to the care plan development, yet they did not participate in the meetings. Their exclusion reflects the hierarchical structure of nursing home care and the belief among many managers that the nursing assistants were not smart enough to contribute. But the larger issue was, once again, chronic under-staffing at the care level. A fully staffed shift meant that there was one nursing assistant assigned to about ten residents. At a bare minimum, each resident needed to be awakened, cleaned, dressed, fed, and assisted in the bathroom. Beds need to be made, household items need to be maintained, and residents need to be kept safe throughout the day. Managers were not willing to take a nursing assistant off the floor, nor were they willing to increase the staff-ing so that they could participate in the fifteen-minute care plan meeting.

The nursing homes were so understaffed that taking one of nursing assistants off the floor posed an unacceptable increased risk that a resident could fall. If the nursing homes had staffed one more nursing assistant to "float" across the units as extra help during the care plan meetings, it would have allowed the nursing homes to access the expertise of nursing assistants, perhaps improving the care plans and increasing the likelihood that they would be followed by the nursing assistants.

Managers and floor staff occupy such different positions in the organizational hierarchy that their understandings of what counts as care have little overlap.[9] Flattening the work hierarchy by including floor staff in the care planning process and requiring managers to work some on the nursing home floor would mitigate organizational conflict. Resident health outcomes improve when nursing assistants are empowered to lend their expertise of direct care in a participatory model of nursing home care.[10] Beyond care, integrating the nursing home workforce into the structure and organization of decision making has been shown to improve workplace satisfaction and lower staff turnover.[11] Indeed, these studies have shown that floor staff want to participate in the care planning process and that when it happens, workers are happier on the job and residents get better care. In fact, recent scholarship has argued that empowering nursing assistants and other direct care workers is essential to reverse the worsening shortage of committed and effective long-term care workers to meet the growing need for care and support services.[12] Similarly, time spent by nurse managers providing direct care on the floor of nursing homes is positively associated with a wide range of better health outcomes.[13] It would also likely alleviate the structural dichotomization between managers and floor staff that creates organizational cultures that generate distrust and suspicion.[14]

In a sense, these conflicts were about negotiating the details of documentation. But they were about more than that. The documentation was a battleground that marked symbolic boundaries between the floor staff and the management. Lamont and Molnar refer to symbolic boundaries as "conceptual distinctions made by social actors to categorize objects, people, practices, and even time and space."[15] People use symbolic resources such as interpretive frames, moral codes, and cultural traditions to construct a set of similarities and differences between themselves and others. In this case, nursing home care workers made attributions of intent about themselves and those above or below them on the organizational hierarchy to mark symbolic boundaries. But the unequal field left the managers with far more power to define the situation, and they exercised that power in a number of ways to enforce the rules about documentation.

It seems reasonable to think that the floor staff and managers would have cooperated because everyone wanted to provide high-quality care. It was the different understandings of what defined that care that were problematic. The discord generated by the documentation was a proxy for control over the conflicting claims of whose work was more important. The floor staff aligned their interests, and their identities, with residents and claimed they did the real, good, and dignified work of caring for people who could not care for themselves.[16] It was possible for nursing assistants to position themselves as "more caring" than managers, and that was how they managed to construct superior identities compared to the managers, because they certainly did not have more authority than them.

4

The Costs of Doing Business

The first three chapters of this book have shown how a range of structural constraints shapes the character of nursing home care work. Medicaid reimbursement and state audits, the health and safety inspections, and the hierarchical battles around the documentation of care exacted an emotional toll, pulling workers in different directions internally and organizationally. Internally, staff members were conflicted about making residents into the embodiment of reimbursable activities. They did what they had to do, but they did not feel good about it. Organizationally, the hierarchy of authority generated animosity and distrust. Managers and floor staff seemed to work in different worlds and with different understandings of the meaning of "care work." This structure provided a context that generated routine conflict and suspicion among workers at both nursing homes. The chronic understaffing in the nursing homes, even when they were "fully staffed," exacerbated the constraints of the reimbursement and regulatory systems. If there were enough staff at the nursing homes, it would not be a problem to supervise all residents while they ate, nor would it be a problem to document and be reimbursed for that care. Further, more staffing would have allowed the nursing assistants the opportunity to leave the floor and join the managers in care plan meetings, creating a stronger basis for mutual recognition and trust.

Both nursing homes were subject to these federal and state policies, and in that sense the distinction between for-profit and nonprofit made little difference. All nursing homes operate in this structure. But that does not mean that all nursing homes behave the same in relation to that structure. Over the course of my fieldwork, the for-profit Golden Bay was winning company awards for profit margins that exceeded expectations while the nonprofit Rolling Hills teetered on the edge of financial ruin. The reasons why, as I explain in this chapter, stem from the different organizational logics of the two nursing homes and their alignment with the reimbursement and regulatory systems. Nursing homes have their own organizational logics that may or may not be consistent with this larger structure. In some cases those logics are aligned and in some cases they are not, and the (mis)alignment between organizational processes and the demands of institutional structures impact the character of work and of workplaces. Sometimes workers resist and other times they acquiesce to the demands of these institutional structures. Golden Bay was broadly consistent in their operations with the types of behaviors that are rewarded financially by the reimbursement system. The managers at Rolling Hills, on the other hand, embraced a logic of institutionalized altruism, which was misaligned with the reimbursement system. Organizational practices around the admissions process, collecting money owed to the facility, and staffing the floors differed between the two facilities. In each case the differences revealed how the reimbursement system rewards behaviors that encourage profit taking and implicitly undermines the mission of nonprofit nursing homes.

Golden Bay did much better than Rolling Hills financially because Golden Bay exemplified the practices that are rewarded by the reimbursement system in the intensely profit driven health care industry, while the mission-oriented Rolling Hills was out of sync with the types of activities that are rewarded by the reimbursement system.[1] When my fieldwork began, Andy and the other managers at Rolling Hills were intentionally mission-oriented. Organizations tell stories about themselves as a means of legitimating themselves to the public, to the state, and to themselves, and Rolling Hills told a mission-minded story.[2] The staff embraced an ethos of institutionalized altruism in their everyday operations. They, at first, acted as a community-oriented facility anchored in nonprofit care, and as such they sought not primarily to make money, but to do good. This was made explicit in various ways to both employees and customers. Their mission statement, for instance, began, "We are a not-for-profit consumer-centered organization committed to meeting the continuing care needs of the aging population in the communities we serve." Their marketing material boasted that "community-service is the hallmark" of the company, and "We believe our nonprofit status comes with a responsibility to provide the community with meaningful, need-driven services." Rolling Hills lived up to that mission in a number of ways. They heavily subsidized a daytime drop-in center for the elderly, sponsored expensive community events during National Nursing Home Week, and organized fund-raisers that integrated the community such as an antique car show and an Iron Chef competition. They participated in the community in other ways, such as taking large groups of residents to the local county fair, and they maintained strong ties to local businesses in the area.

The managers at Golden Bay were more concerned about being a successful business than they were about community service. Golden Bay's mission statement reflected that orientation: "With quality care as our bottom line, we strive each day to surpass all expectations in how we serve our customers." The financial metaphor of a "bottom line" and referring to residents as "customers" signify a business orientation to nursing home care that was much different from that of the mission-oriented Rolling Hills. The company's bullet-pointed list of "core values" included "Employees are the company, Quality care is our bottom line, Surpass all expectations, Ownership and accountability," and finally "Serve the customer." It was clearly business oriented, and the managers at Golden Bay were committed to the financial success of the nursing home. Golden Bay's corporate offices reinforced that narrative, peppering the nursing home with articles, pamphlets, tip sheets, and conference call meetings that reviewed strategies to enhance revenue streams and cut costs. They also recognized the nursing home with awards for surpassing revenue expectations.

At the start of my fieldwork, the two nursing homes engaged in different practices along three key dimensions—admissions, collecting money owed by residents, and staffing. Golden Bay prioritized Medicare beneficiaries in the admissions process and then extended their stay in the facility as long as they could, aggressively collected money owed to the nursing home, and kept labor costs low by refusing to use temporary staffing agencies to fill vacant shifts. In contrast, Rolling Hills took a "first-come, first-served" approach to admissions, allowed residents to slide on money owed to the facility, and got caught up in a pattern of extensive use of staffing agencies to fill vacant shifts. In each case, Rolling Hills at first made decisions from an altruistic orientation.

By the middle of my fieldwork, these more altruistic practices got Rolling Hills into financial trouble. As it got worse, Andy and his staff abandoned to a considerable extent their mission orientation and engaged in business practices that were consistent with what Golden Bay did. Organizations have the tendency to become more similar, especially in times of uncertainty and crisis. This process, called institutional isomorphism, was for Rolling Hills a matter of organizational survival.[3] Andy directed his staff to engage in the kind of profit-driven business practices that he said drove him to the nonprofit sector in the first place. By the end of my fieldwork, Andy was relieved of his duties as administrator and was replaced with a new administrator who was firmly oriented toward repairing the financial standing of Rolling Hills.

Managing Admissions

Nursing homes need to carefully manage their admissions process because Medicaid residents reimburse a lot less and stay a lot longer than Medicare and self-pay residents. Lucy, the director of nursing at Golden Bay, explained this: "There is a balance. Like, the building could not function on Medicaid alone. We couldn't pay our bills. We don't get reimbursed enough and the state keeps taking more and more money away. We could not stay open. The building would close. So we have to have the Medicare, commercial insurance, and the private [self-pay] in order to pay the rest of the Medicaid bills." For this reason, when she and Cynthia took over the organizational leadership of the nursing home they prioritized Medicare over Medicaid. Cynthia explained, "Pushing out the Medicare rate was the first thing. Something that—pushing up the Medicare census a little bit is something that we worked on." She monitored the numbers closely. Cynthia said, "We do a lot of projections, so—I have spreadsheets that I use that I put in every expense; how much we're spending for nursing supplies, how much labor we're using, everything, and you get a bottom line. And so, that's something that I monitor. When you see us go to Kirsten's [rehabilitation coordinator] office, what I'm getting out of that is what's our Medicare rate gonna be?" They boosted Medicare revenue by increasing the number of Medicare residents they admitted, extending the length of stay for each Medicare resident, and building up the rehabilitation and restorative services offered by the facility, since Medicare reimburses nursing homes only for short-term rehabilitation after a qualifying three-night hospital stay.

Cynthia, Lucy, and Francine, the admissions coordinator, tightly controlled the admissions process at Golden Bay. Cynthia was a careful person, and I could tell that in our interview she was actively monitoring her presentation of self. She explained that Golden Bay does not discriminate against Medicaid beneficiaries, saying emphatically, "We truly do take all people! You're supposed to and I know a lot of places don't. We'll take straight Medicaid. That's expensive for us but I feel it's our civic duty and you're not supposed to discriminate on payer source." Yet in the year and a half I spent doing fieldwork there, despite Cynthia's assertion, the admissions decisions unambiguously favored Medicare beneficiaries who required expensive rehabilitation services related to orthopedic surgeries like a hip or knee replacement. Francine carefully admitted that "Medicaid is sort of last on the list, but it's—we don't deny them." Lucy was candid: "I'm not going to take a custodial person into a Medicare, high-paying bed and have them sit there for the next ten years when I could roll the bed over every three or four weeks."

The high reimbursement rates of the Medicare program combined with the quick turnover of residents made for a clear preference to the low reimbursement rates of the Medicaid program for beneficiaries who could live at the facility for years before they died. Lucy explained, "When I'm looking at residents to go on the rehab unit, I'm going to look at people that have either Medicare or commercial insurance. If I have an open bed [on the long-term care unit], I'm going to take a custodial person [whose care is paid by Medicaid or, more preferably, out of pocket]."

Medicare residents were in high demand and short supply. The reason why is they reimburse a lot more than Medicaid or self-pay residents and they have much faster "turnover" in that residents stay for weeks instead of years. To most effectively access and leverage Medicare reimbursements, a rehabilitation gym staffed with physical, occupational, and speech therapists helps the facility make more money because they can bill Medicare for these skilled services. Furthermore, a program of "restorative care" designed to restore a resident's abilities, such as eating independently, also is part of the Medicare reimbursement system. Golden Bay excelled in these areas compared to Rolling Hills. Golden Bay's rehabilitation gym was staffed seven days a week by approximately a dozen therapists, compared to that at Rolling Hills, which had a few therapists and operated five days a week. Golden Bay had an active restorative care program and Rolling Hills did not. In addition to staffing these high-reimbursing services, Golden Bay also marketed them effectively compared to Rolling Hills.

Francine explained that the Golden Bay corporate office "will call and say, you know, I need this, I need that, I need this. Medicare is down so they want to know what we're doing to, you know, get Medicare." She explained that her supervisors expected that she "do marketing every day." She marketed the facility to potential residents in the community by trying to draw them inside Golden Bay so they could see that there was nothing to fear. She organized a variety of events, including a martini bar with a guest speaker who gave a presentation about what to look for when shopping for a nursing home. Francine also brought prospective residents to the facility with an invited speaker from AARP, who discussed driving for elders. She also planned an event for people who had home care or were in assisted living to visit the facility. Overall the pressure from corporate to market and promote the facility was a daily burden on Francine, and she was upset that they expected her to call individuals for an explanation why they chose to go to competing nursing homes. "I think that's wrong. It's their own personal business," she explained. In addition to marketing to potential residents, Golden Bay also promoted their rehabilitation services directly to orthopedic surgeons at the nearest regional hospital.

Hospital staff are not supposed to provide recommendations about specific nursing homes to patients, but Francine's hospital liaison, Anne, spent several days per week in hospitals cultivating a network of physicians and social workers who referred patients for nursing home services. She organized tours of the rehabilitation gym so hospital staff could view it, hoping they would direct patients to the facility. Judged by Golden Bay's strong financial performance, this seemed to be a successful marketing strategy.

Rather than build a customer base by courting orthopedists like Golden Bay, Rolling Hills had "screeners" in hospitals who worked on commission to place patients in need of rehabilitation in the facility. When the screeners found a suitable candidate, they sent the information to Beverly, the admissions coordinator, who reviewed referrals and shared them with Joanne and the unit managers, and then made a decision about whether to accept or reject. Rolling Hills' turnaround time from referral to a decision was several days, notably slower than that of Golden Bay, which was only hours. Rolling Hills' marketing plan also included their sponsorship of a community elderly day center in the nearby town, where elderly folks could drop in at anytime during the day. The center provided social support, various activities, and food to these individuals. Every week, Liz or Flo, the dietary manager, drove to the center with boxes of food to serve to the elders. It was a crucial piece of Rolling Hills' commitment to its surrounding community, but it was also a significant financial expense. It did, however, bring in business, although likely too many of the wrong kind of residents (Medicaid) because working-class and low-income elderly individuals were most likely to use the drop-in center and then come to Rolling Hills when they required care.

Golden Bay did a better job than Rolling Hills at recruiting Medicare residents. Golden Bay also went to great lengths to extend their length of stay in the facility as long as possible. Kirsten was an occupational therapist who had recently been promoted to rehabilitation services manager. In our interview, she explained, "The whole goal supposedly for the company is to have a longer length of stay and treat for shorter minutes because that's what they think is appropriate. But it's really just because that's how they can make more money." She said that the company wanted her to lower the amount of daily rehabilitation her department provided to residents:

KIRSTEN: The company's saying that we're overdelivering rehab and I need to control it better by taking away some therapy. Because, as I have been reminded several times when I've had this argument, we are *not* a not-for-profit organization. We are here to make money and if we're giving treatment that we're not getting paid for then we're not making money.

JASON: What is that like to hear?

KIRSTEN: It totally pisses me off and I feel bad because I feel like I'm getting to be used to it enough that it doesn't bother me as much anymore. 'Cause it used to really bother me and now I'm, well, we just don't have a choice. And I think that kind of sucks because I really want to be a patient advocate, and get them what they need and what's clinically appropriate. But on the other hand when I'm supposed to be in here telling the therapists, "You're not gonna have a job if we don't make money because we're over-treating everybody," it's hard for me to balance that out.

Kirsten clashed often with Barbara, the clinical case manager in charge of Medicare reimbursement. The tensions they experienced between the logic of cost and the logic of care were often latent but occasionally they erupted openly. At the daily managers meeting, for instance, when the social worker explained that a Medicare resident had completed his rehabilitation and was preparing to be discharged, Barbara interjected swiftly, "But we're not ready to discharge." She explained that "it would be great to keep him until Friday," which would allow the facility to bill Medicare for extra covered days of care. Lucy agreed it would be great to hold him, but said with a snicker that it might be tough because "he walked into the shower today with his clothes under his arm," meaning he was obviously healthy enough to go home. Cynthia argued that extending his stay would benefit him because "he's really into it [rehabilitation]" and "we can say we're working on his endurance." Kirsten, who had notified the social worker that the resident was strong enough to go home, turned to Barbara and coldly stated, "Well I'm not going to lie." Barbara responded brusquely, "I'm not asking you to lie."

I asked Barbara about the conflict later that morning. As she showed me the company's written expectations for Medicare utilization, she explained, "My biggest pressure is to try to keep rehab from sending them home." She pointed out that the company expected the average length of stay for Medicare residents to be forty days. Their average at the time was thirty-six days. A few years earlier, "the company was losing money hand over fist," said Barbara, "and they came down on the clinical case managers and asked us to take charge of the care of Medicare residents" instead of the rehabilitation department and the social workers, who advocated for residents to go home as soon as clinically appropriate.

The management at Rolling Hills did not engage in this practice, even though Andy seemed occasionally tempted. For example, one morning Beverly announced that the census had dipped to 90 percent of capacity.

Jamie, the lead social worker, stated at the morning meeting that four residents were ready to go home. Andy quipped, "We're at 90 percent, they're not ready to go home yet!" And as the staff chuckled he added, "Just kidding." Andy's joke seemed to represent anxiety about the low census, and perhaps a desire to extend the stay of those residents, but to the best of my knowledge it never occurred. It was no wonder Golden Bay won awards for their Medicare reimbursement and Rolling Hills contended with rising deficits.

The practices I observed, in which Golden Bay but not Rolling Hills gamed Medicare as much as possible without crossing the fraud line, is consistent with the findings of a recent study conducted by the Office of Inspector General of the Department of Health and Human Services, revealingly titled *Questionable Billing by Skilled Nursing Facilities*.[4] The Office of Inspector General found that from 2006 to 2008, for-profit nursing homes were significantly more likely than nonprofit nursing homes to bill Medicare for the highest reimbursement rate category.[5] Of Medicare residents in for-profit facilities, 32 percent were classified in the highest daily payment category, compared to 18 percent for nonprofits and 13 percent for state-owned facilities. For-profit facilities also kept Medicare residents for an average of twenty-nine days, substantially longer than the twenty-three-day average at nonprofits. These differences, the report found, "were not the result of differences in beneficiary populations," meaning that for-profits and nonprofits serve individuals with similar care needs, but for-profits are billing more and holding residents longer than nonprofits.[6] The largest for-profit nursing home chains, such as the chain that Golden Bay was a part of, were the most likely to bill Medicare at the highest possible rate and to extend the stay of residents. The report concluded, "These billing patterns indicate that certain [skilled nursing facilities] may be routinely placing beneficiaries into higher paying [reimbursement categories] regardless of the beneficiaries' care and resource needs or keeping beneficiaries in [Medicare] Part A stays longer than necessary."[7]

Andy occasionally told me that for every nursing home in the black, two or three were in the red. Perhaps this was a way for him to save face because it is clear that the nursing home industry is quite profitable. The Medicare Payment Advisory Commission (MedPAC) reported that in 2009, the average Medicare profit margin for nursing homes was over 18 percent. In fact, MedPAC reported for seven consecutive years that the aggregate profit margins in free-standing nursing homes exceeded 10 percent.[8] Medicare payments are a key piece of generating margins. The clearest path to profitability is in optimizing the balance among Medicare, private payers, and commercial insurance residents to offset the lower Medicaid payments.

Andy was by no means naïve about the economics of long-term care, and he said he was proud to make money for the company. But he intended to do so using a logic of institutionalized altruism rather than cost efficiency, a key reason why he came to Rolling Hills. Consistent with this logic, Beverly admitted residents on a first-come, first-served basis with little inclination to discriminate based on payer source. She was fairly new as the admissions coordinator, but had spent the previous ten years as the manager of the rehabilitation unit. About a month after I began fieldwork, I walked into her office as she sat at her desk. It was a busy day; she had a half dozen referrals under consideration. On the wall behind her was a large diagram of the facility, with a list of who occupied each room, color coded by payer type. I counted eleven Medicare residents, well below the budget, which called for twenty. With every referral, Beverly said she considered a range of factors, including whether the individual had stayed at Rolling Hills before, if a family member was or had been a resident, the individual's overall health status, and whether she felt the resident would be a good fit for the unit. Ultimately this way of admitting residents, filling the beds while largely ignoring the payer source, led to the facility's budget crisis. Reimbursement systems do not necessarily favor for-profit facilities over nonprofits; rather, they favor particular types of activities. Rolling Hills made admissions decisions that were consistent with the kind of nursing home they wanted to be, but that was also inconsistent with what the reimbursement system rewards, until it became clear the nursing home was on the brink of financial ruin.

I interviewed Beverly, the admissions coordinator at Rolling Hills, and I asked her about their admissions process. She was in her sixties, with graying hair, glasses, and a thick New England accent. She explained that at first she was "census driven" and "I wanted to fill the beds." Andy supported that; he wanted a full house, and it was consistent with the community-oriented mission of a nonprofit nursing home. However, it quickly generated an unfavorable case mix and problematic financial projections. The census was filled with too many Medicaid residents and not enough Medicare. Rolling Hills was budgeted to have twenty Medicare residents in-house daily, but through the spring and summer months the Medicare census often fluctuated between ten and fourteen and got as low as six, which Andy called "scary" and explained to me that "there's no way to make a profit when it's that low." Moreover, the rehabilitation unit, where Medicare residents are supposed to stay, was nearly full of long-term Medicaid residents. These individuals could be on the unit for years, even though they were likely a better fit for the other units.

Andy confided in me that his supervisor, Mike, was concerned about the nursing home's finances. Through the long hot summer of 2007, Andy faced mounting pressure from Mike to raise Medicare income and better contain expenses. Mike began to make weekly visits to the facility. The corporate office also held weekly marketing meetings with Andy and Beverly, which were specifically intended to boost Medicare. Supervisors also visited Rolling Hills to check the Medicare reimbursement claims that Carol submitted. They wanted to double-check that she had claimed all the Medicare reimbursement money possible given the case mix. Carol told me in her dry, sarcastic style, "I can't turn eight Medicare patients into eighteen." Andy was upbeat publicly, but privately he fretted over the budget's "aggressive Medicare projections." Carol thought that perhaps the low Medicare census reflected little more than the seasonality of their business: Medicare numbers go up in the winter because elders are prone to slip on ice or snow and fracture a hip or clavicle. In the summer, fewer people have elective surgeries that require lengthy and expensive rehabilitation. That seems reasonable and may be correct, but by the time the summer turned to autumn, it was clear there were bigger problems afoot.

Andy asked Carol to call their nearby competitors and gauge if others were down on Medicare. Carol reported back that the other facilities seemed to be doing better than Rolling Hills. "It was killing us," Beverly said about the case mix. She continued, "So at that point, the pressure was, you know, 'we need to send these people home.' We lost a lot of people, we sent some people home, we moved some people and freed up rooms on our units." Determined to improve the case mix, Andy became increasingly vigilant about opening beds intended for Medicare payers.

Bed Management

Rolling Hills had a problem. The beds typically reserved for Medicare residents on the rehabilitation unit were filled with Medicaid residents. They wanted to move those individuals to the long-term care unit or the dementia unit, but the 1987 Nursing Home Reform Act required permission from residents or family members before they could do so. At the morning meeting, Andy discussed his desire to change a resident's room despite the family's objections. Andy said the resident was "inappropriately placed on the rehab unit," and Liz, the activities director, added, "At the family's request." Andy continued, "And we think she should be on the dementia unit. I've left a few messages with the daughter and said if you do not respond in forty-eight hours we are moving her. The family responded and said no. But I'm going to call the daughter again with our rationale." Andy's public rationale was that the scope of care on the dementia unit was more appropriate than the rehabilitation unit. That was correct, but in his backstage rationale with the staff, he directed them to "take Beverly's lead, she's trying to open up Medicare beds, and this is the worst month we've had for those. The beds are full, but we have five or six Medicare people and the operation is grinding to a halt."

Beverly had a handful of unoccupied beds on the dementia unit; they were the most difficult beds to fill. Prospective residents' families were scared of the unit or resisted because they could not bring themselves to admit that their loved one had dementia. Beverly approached several residents who lived on the rehabilitation unit and asked them to relocate to the dementia unit, but they refused. Those families were already familiar with the unit's staff and did not want to take a chance with staff on a new unit. Jamie, the lead social worker, described the difficulties involved: "Sometimes it's a hard sell to get people to go down to the dementia unit, even though they might really need it because they're cognitively impaired and the activities down there are much more appropriate. It can be safer for them with a large unit, but the families cannot accept the idea that mom or dad's got dementia."

Misplaced residents affected the staff as well as the residents. Cindy, the nursing assistant who was "reamed out" by her supervisor in the previous chapter, said she liked to work on the rehabilitation unit because she found satisfaction in caring for people who started in a wheelchair then progressed to a walker and then proceeded out the door and back home. But she was increasingly stuck taking care of individuals with advanced dementia. One morning as I approached Cindy to help her pass out breakfast trays, she turned to me and said, "We have a lot of behaviors this morning" and said that Neddie, a resident, had thrown her commode at another resident. Cindy said, "I don't need to tell you what happened next," and I must have looked perplexed because she explained, "Shit went all over the floor." Cindy also told me, "I have five or six residents on my hall that should be on the dementia unit!" and it seriously impeded her workflow. "This is not my job!" she said. In her view, her job was to help individuals recover from injuries, not help them remember their names.

As the financial picture became increasingly bleak, Andy and Beverly asked Liz, the activities director, to give residents and families whose rooms they wanted to change a sales pitch. She was gregarious, a jokester who entertained residents and made them laugh. She appeared to have genuine emotional connections to many residents. She had been on staff for many years and was very well acquainted with the concerns residents and their families have about nursing homes and especially the dementia unit. Liz also was persuasive; she gave tours to families and had some success moving residents. But sometimes she used dubious methods. One morning I sat in the conference room and chatted with Liz as we waited for the daily meeting to begin. The manager of the rehabilitation unit, Dawn, walked into the room. Liz stood up and approached Dawn and the two high-fived. Liz said victoriously, "My plan worked!" They were talking about her plan to move a resident off Dawn's unit. The resident refused initially, and then Liz came up with the idea of moving a dying resident into her room, in the hopes that it would change her mind. It did.

Rolling Hills aggressively sought ways to open up beds available for Medicare beneficiaries. Bed management was one of Andy's most important operational and financial management tools and is a hidden means of stratifying nursing home residents. Medicaid residents are moved around the facility to accommodate Medicare and self-payers. This is another mechanism in which residents suffer the effects of being treated as the embodiment of reimbursable activities.

The staff at Golden Bay occasionally asked residents to change rooms, but they did not need to be as aggressive in this matter as Rolling Hills became. From the point of admission, they were more careful about placing residents on the most appropriate unit. Susan, the lead social worker at Golden Bay, did not appreciate the occasions when the staff asked residents to move because it seemed to benefit only the facility. An experienced social worker, she challenged her colleagues when they sought a room change. At the daily managers meeting, Lucy told the managers that a resident was moved to a new room, but had not been informed prior to the room change, even though her legal guardian had approved it. Lucy relayed the events to the managers at the morning meeting and said, sympathetically, "She thought she did something wrong." Lucy said it was a "big deal" and that the managers must communicate better about these issues. Susan agreed but added, "We have got to do better than that; she was really upset!" She continued, "We've got to do better, I mean, it is for our convenience that we ask people to change rooms." She restated for emphasis, "It is for our convenience." Her colleague played the role of peacemaker: "And that's okay, as long as we have the consent of the guardian or the resident." Lucy agreed, but added, "From now on, we have got to overdo it, make sure that we overdo it and tell the resident." Later in the day I asked Susan about bed management. She said, "Switching rooms. You know, I do understand there is an upper level everywhere and regional people are telling care people. But I try to be fair. I tell the families 'It's a nice room or it's not, or it's close to the nurses' station,' I try to work with them. I try to work for both sides." As an experienced social worker, Susan understood the financial dimension but said her role was to strike a balance and be an advocate for residents' rights. "How far do you push it for advocacy of people's rights?" she asked rhetorically.

Collecting Debts

After residents were admitted to the facility, there was the matter of collecting payment. This was another area in which Golden Bay excelled and Rolling Hills lagged. While Rolling Hills at first allowed residents time to pay their bills when they could, Golden Bay collected payments aggressively. Golden Bay's billing office was just past the front foyer, first door on the left, and staffed with three employees. Dan, Golden Bay's billing manager, a short, wiry gentleman in his early sixties, described the billing department as "the nucleus" and "the heartbeat" of the facility. Dan was responsible to collect money owed to the facility by Medicaid, Medicare, or commercial insurance companies, while Ruby, his colleague and the financial manager, worked to collect outstanding balances from individuals. When Ruby took the job initially, she felt uncomfortable calling families about the money they owed the facility. But those feelings changed as she got used to the requirements of the position. She got comfortable with the idea of care as a commodity, explaining to me, "If you're asking for money that maybe you aren't completely entitled to I would feel awkward, but in this case when I have to call families or residents, you know—if you provide the service, if you bought something at J. C. Penney and you have it in your possession and you're wearing it, then you should pay for it. So that's basically the way that I look at it." She was proud that her collection rate was over 90 percent and claimed it was better than the rates at most nursing homes. She even boasted that she could teach the "young MBAs at corporate" how to collect money efficiently. Ruby's experience in retail prior to the nursing home care industry may explain how she thought of nursing care: a simple market exchange, no different from buying clothes at a department store.

While Ruby had integrated market ideology into her practice of nursing home care, Janet, her counterpart at Rolling Hills, had a far more difficult time reconciling care as if it was a business transaction. Collecting debts was difficult emotionally for Janet; she empathized with families who could not afford to pay. The persistence of an ethic of care that highlighted compassion and altruism clouded the budgetary demands upon which the facility foundered. One morning I wandered down the main hallway and saw Janet, the financial manager at Rolling Hills. She was standing outside Andy's office. She turned to me and announced, "It's time for my monthly slap-down!" The accounts receivables meeting with her corporate supervisors was about to begin. Andy invited me to sit in and observe the meeting with his supervisors, who participated by speakerphone. Andy, Janet, and Charlotte, who handled medical records, gathered in Andy's small office, around a circular table that held a large red binder labeled "AR 2007." Inside the binder was the detailed financial information and payment history of every resident.

On the conference call, Andy and Janet's company supervisors went through a list of about fifteen residents with outstanding balances, some of them having accumulated for several months. The supervisors asked them to explain what they had done to collect since the previous month's call. As Janet and the supervisors went through the list, Andy explained to Charlotte how the system works. With the binder open, and within my view, he taught us, "This is the money we haven't collected yet. We want these all zeroes" as he motioned to numbers on the page. "We want to collect as soon as possible." He warned about lawyers who hid assets to make it appear as if residents could not afford to pay for their care and thus qualify for Medicaid benefits fraudulently. Andy complained that it is bad for the facility, and that "I don't want to gouge people's life savings, but people should pay for their care. Instead of getting two hundred sixty dollars a day [the cost for private payers] we get one hundred ten [a low Medicaid reimbursement]. Then we got revenue problems."

Indeed, Rolling Hills got revenue problems. Terse and churlish, the supervising voices on the phone gave the impression Janet had done a poor job, but also that she could never do enough. When they discussed Harriet, a resident who owed the facility about five thousand dollars, the supervisor asked simply, "Can we get any more from her?" Janet said that the facility could take only half her monthly personal funds paid by Medicaid, a paltry thirty dollars a month. Another resident had an outstanding balance of six thousand dollars. They asked Janet, "Did you ask her about income?" Janet, her tone of voice somewhere between acquiescence and disgust, explained, "She's on hospice," strongly implying that given her delicate health condition, inquiring about her income would be inappropriate. The woman's voice on the phone shot back, "But we need income. We could lose six thousand dollars." Janet said a Medicaid application had been submitted. Corporate told Janet, "We need proof the application has been submitted because Medicaid hasn't registered it, and if the family can't prove it, we'll need to start discharge. I know that's aggressive, but we've lost six thousand dollars." The highest debt owed to Rolling Hills was fourteen thousand dollars. The voice on the phone told Janet to "call the daughter and suggest we be her representative payee. No. Tell her. I'm being polite. Say we need the money, fourteen thousand dollars right away."

The meeting ended after one of the supervisors asked Janet to follow up on the "three worst accounts" and report back via email by the day's close of business. One of those accounts was Marlene's ten thousand dollar debt. Andy asked Janet to get Marlene; he wanted to speak with her. In the meantime he explained to me that he had been "way too aggressive with Medicare projections" and it threw off the entire budget. In 2006 Rolling Hills budgeted for 14 percent of their total beds designated for Medicare residents and increased it to 17 percent for 2007. They rarely reached even half that amount. By comparison, Golden Bay budgeted for 15.5 percent of their beds filled with Medicare payers both years and typically met their budget.

Marlene propelled her wheelchair to Andy's office. As she pulled into his doorway she said with a forlorn resignation, "I was expecting this." A checkbook and a copy of her bill were wedged between her thigh and the wheelchair. Andy patted her knee lightly and reassured her, "Don't worry," and explained, "everything will be straightened out but we need good, accurate information from you." Andy asked to see Marlene's bill. When he looked at it, it was too complicated for even him to interpret. He put down the bill and asked if Marlene had submitted an application for Medicaid. She said that it was sent in several months ago but had not been approved because her husband refused to send the deed to their house. He feared the state would take their house away. Andy assured Marlene that would not happen and volunteered to call her husband to reiterate. He reassured her several times that there was nothing to worry about and that he was not going to kick her out of the nursing home. Yet in the next breath he explained that if she did not yet qualify for Medicaid, the expenses since the application was submitted would be transferred to Marlene's private balance. Marlene left Andy's office, wheeled to the business office, and then wrote a check for a few thousand dollars to the facility.

Andy said Janet should have never allowed these debts to get so large. He told me that Rolling Hills ranked second worst in the company for the length of time to collect payment and added, "I don't need my boss telling me that the financial coordinator is reading the newspaper for forty-five minutes." He demoted Janet to a receptionist position a few weeks later but hoped she would quit instead (she did, and called her demotion "humiliating"). Andy promoted Charlotte to financial coordinator. I interviewed Charlotte about a month after she took the position, when she explained, "Corporate is up there, you know, pointing their finger and, you know, 'gotta get that money,' so—they don't deal with the people coming in, and you know, they don't have to deal with them face-to-face. They're just looking at numbers on a page saying, you know, 'we're owed this, you need to collect this, this, this, and this, and this is what you need to do.'" I asked if she planned to stay in the position, and she said, "I did not ask for this job. I was told 'this is your new role, or there's the door.'"

Staffing

The financial problems at Rolling Hills were exacerbated by a sharp increase in labor expenses that Andy would have to reign in if he intended to keep his job. Both nursing homes held to the industry standard nursing ratios of one nursing assistant for ten residents and one nurse for twenty residents, give or take a few residents depending on the day, but there was an important difference in staffing as Rolling Hills used agency staffing to fill vacancies in the schedule. Private agencies hire nursing assistants and nurses, and the agencies contract with health services organizations such as nursing homes and then provide staff to the nursing homes as needed. Utilizing staffing agencies was expensive and brought in staff of unknown quality to the nursing home, but on the plus side the shifts were filled. Golden Bay had not utilized agency staffing for more than three years. When they had openings on the schedule, managers themselves worked on the floor or else mandated an employee who had worked the previous shift to stay on for the next shift.

Cynthia explained to me that when she became the administrator of Golden Bay, one of her top priorities was to eliminate agency staffing from the nursing home. In our interview, she went on at length about how before she started the facility "couldn't make money because they were using so much agency" and warned that sometimes nursing homes use so much that they become so reliant on staffing agencies that the building cannot operate without them. This was an oblique reference to Andy at Rolling Hills. She and Andy knew I was doing research at both facilities. She contrasted her success at Golden Bay with what was happening at Rolling Hills: "We are a successful building but if you can't support yourself and you can't make money, you won't survive. And you've seen what happens to administrators who can't make that happen, even if it's a good building and you're doing a good job otherwise." She was proud to have not utilized agency staff for more than three years, and it was clear that neither she nor Lucy had any interest in using them ever again. I was told that agency staff often cost double the total labor costs of in-house staff. Agency nurses get paid substantially more per hour than in-house staff, and the referral agency collects a per-shift fee from the facility.[9]

The issue of whether to use agency staffing divided the floor staff and the management at Golden Bay. Some of the nursing assistants and nurses were angry that the managers mandated them to stay after their shift ended instead of utilizing nurse staffing agencies to fill vacancies. Tensions boiled over at an all-staff meeting that I observed. Staff members gathered in the main dining room; Cynthia stood in front of a big easel with a large pad that noted the meeting's agenda. She intended to review the results of an employee satisfaction survey, which yielded generally positive results. Her brief presentation finished with a wide-open, provocative question: "Does anyone have anything they want to say?"

The first question regarded pay raises, and a brief debate ensued about whether all staff should get the same percentage raise or whether it should vary by performance or job tenure. Carissa sat a few seats from me. I watched her become increasingly agitated until she raised her hand and then interjected loudly. She decried the mandated staffing policy at Golden Bay, called it "insulting" and "demeaning" and said it is symbolically "telling me that my outside life is worthless." Rather than allowing staff members to go home when their shift ended, she said, they are forced to be "angry at work." A nursing aide added from the back, "A happy staff makes for happy residents."[10] Carissa closed with, "We need to look at other staffing options," and although she did not explicitly say to use agency staff, that was what she meant. Cynthia retorted that mandated staffing comes with the territory of health care work and that all the health care organizations she had ever worked for mandated staff to stay after their shift. She explained that she could not allow staff members to leave if it would put residents' safety at risk. High turnover of nursing assistants, which by some measurements reaches 100 percent annually, accounts for a great deal of the reason why the vast majority of nursing homes utilize staffing agencies.[11]

Phoebe, a nursing assistant, raised a related issue: too many of her colleagues called out sick and left others to carry the load. She liked Golden Bay's "no fault" call-out policy, but asked, "Can't something be done [about staff members who abuse the policy]?" Gia, the human resources manager, told Phoebe and Carissa to blame their coworkers for mandated staffing because "they are the ones who call out when it's a sunny day." Cynthia argued that staff members were not mandated often, and when they were, it was typically for only a half hour. A nursing assistant countered, "Every day in this building at least one CNA is mandated to stay" and said it was often for four hours. Carissa declared, "Just once is enough" and said that in nursing homes that use agency staff there is typically no mandating of in-house staff. Cynthia tepidly defended herself: "I can't change the system." Then she

turned to Carissa and told her, "If you are not going to be able to work somewhere that has mandated staffing, then maybe this job isn't for you. I know
that's harsh, but that's the reality."

Just after the meeting ended, I walked into Cynthia's office. She sat behind
her desk, gave me an exasperated look, sighed, and said, "That did not go
well." She maintained that nurses are not mandated to stay very often, but
that when they are, it is part of the job of being a nurse. "It happens everywhere," she said, and added, "There's no way we're bringing in agency." Clearly
unhappy with how the staff meeting unfolded, her long day was about to get
longer: she got up from her desk and said, "Okay, now I have to go talk with
an irate family member who is threatening to sue us for millions of dollars."

Cynthia and Lucy said that agency staff were too expensive and that
they had no investment in the facility's success, no knowledge of the residents, and no interest in work outside of their paycheck. They were not
emotionally invested in the residents. Gia, for example, said, "The level of
care is not as good because [agency staff] don't care." She said the quality of
care had gone up since the nursing home stopped using agency three years
ago. Lucy summed up her views on the matter when she explained to me,
"When you bring agency into the building, they don't; for one thing, they
have no loyalty to the company or to the building. They have no loyalty to
the residents. They're just here to do a job and collect their eight hours and
that's that."

Not all managers agreed with Cynthia and Lucy. Crystal for one had a different point of view on agency staffing. As a manager, she was on call every
third weekend and the nursing home had chronic difficulty staffing the facility on weekends. In response to Lucy's point of view on agency, she said,
"Lucy's pretty removed when its two o'clock on Saturday afternoon and half
the staff is leaving because they're only scheduled six o'clock to two o'clock
and you're faced with mandating them again or trying to pick amongst them
who should be mandated. Is it the person who's been here for sixteen hours
already or is it the person who's got a three-year-old at home that they've
gotta get back to?"

Andy knew Golden Bay well, and when I told Andy that Golden Bay had
not used agency in more than three years, he rolled his eyes and said, "Well,
they can get away with that because they don't protect their managers." He
was right. The managers at Golden Bay were much more likely to work on
the floor on weekends because they did not have enough staff. I observed
numerous Thursday afternoons when the managers called staff members
to ask if they could cover the weekend shift. They offered bonuses to full-
time staff to work extra shifts, but a lot of times they worked on the floor

themselves because they could not get enough people to work during their scheduled days off.

Cynthia said she was reluctant to use agency staff because "the more you use, sometimes the more entrenched you get." She knew that this became a problem for Andy at Rolling Hills. After a handful of full-time nursing assistants and nurses resigned or were fired in the spring of 2007, the nursing home began to rely heavily on staffing agencies to cover scheduling vacancies. This sudden and unanticipated increase in labor expenses exacerbated the already difficult financial picture at Rolling Hills.

Every Thursday, Andy completed a staffing report and emailed it to his boss, Mike. This report specified the number of labor hours used, the cost, and the percentage of those hours filled by staffing agencies. In December 2007 Andy showed me the summary staffing report for the entire year. It revealed a massive spike in agency use that began in the middle of 2007. In the first few months of 2007, Rolling Hills used about sixty hours of nursing assistant agency staffing per week and around forty hours of licensed nursing staff. In May 2007 both began to rise dramatically. Andy said he was "getting killed on agency," and all of a sudden the floors were staffed with around one hundred fifty hours of nursing assistant agency staffing and about eighty hours of licensed nursing agency staffing every week. Considering the budget called for zero hours of nursing agency use, the huge increase in agency staffing severely damaged the facility's financial picture. By the end of 2007, the nursing assistant agency staffing had declined somewhat, but remained over a hundred hours per week for every week through the end of the year, while licensed nursing agency use fluctuated between fifty and eighty hours.

In the past, Rolling Hills had offered a free CNA training course with the promise of full-time employment if the trainees passed the certification exam. They had success hiring staff with this program, but Andy had passed on organizing this program in the spring of 2007, just before the spike in agency usage. Now he wondered aloud to himself, "What was I thinking?" He tried to find staff through traditional means, placing classified ads in local newspapers and on radio stations. Andy was unwilling to have the facility operate chronically short on staff and preferred to have shifts fully covered, even with agency staff.

The huge increase in agency utilization affected all three units, but none more than the rehabilitation unit. Dawn described it as a "clinical unit" because there are frequent changes to doctors' orders and special instructions from rehabilitation specialists that must be followed.[12] The unit also managed the nerves of anxious family members who were restless to bring their loved ones home. I interviewed Dawn, the unit's manager, a week before she resigned to take a position at a nearby nursing home. She described the dearth of permanent staff on her unit as "one of my biggest annoyances in this building." The unit is "ever-changing," and agency staff "are not invested in what happens. There is no way to hold them accountable. Or teach them. But I have a yearly survey to deal with."

Tina was responsible for scheduling staff at Rolling Hills and was deeply involved in the hiring process. Andy instructed her to hire new nursing aides and use part-time staff more often, but neither seemed to materialize. High agency usage continued, and several staff members became suspicious of Tina. There were persistent rumors that Tina held a second job at the agency that routinely sent nursing staff to the facility. Moonlighting at the agency, if true, would have been an obvious conflict of interest. Some staff members even suggested Tina received bonuses whenever the agency's staff worked at Rolling Hills.

The pressure on Andy got intense. He had the feeling his days were numbered when Mike began to visit the facility every week. Staffing became a frequent topic of conversation at the managers meetings. Andy told them, "Every hour of CNA agency is a severe operational challenge for Mike." He added, "This is the most consistent pressure on revenue we have, and I haven't moved the needle on that. I am being graded on that, and I am failing." He revealed that the nursing home was spending ten thousand dollars per month on agency staff, and it had lost a half million dollars in 2007. He told me privately, "I may not be here in ninety days. I have to think about the long-term health of the facility." In a last-ditch effort, Andy announced that he would hold each manager responsible for recruiting one nursing assistant a week until they got labor costs under control. A few days later, Mike fired Andy.

Few staff members were surprised when Andy was let go. Andy himself was not surprised. Offhand remarks to several managers and me implied that he knew it was coming. The managers learned of Andy's fate from Mike. He told them that as much as he liked Andy personally, he was given numerous opportunities to improve the facility's performance, and at this point there was no choice other than to let him go. Several months later, Cynthia ran into Andy at a professional conference. Andy told her that the company was not satisfied with Rolling Hills' financial performance. He reportedly told her, "I couldn't get away from agency." Although Andy and I had very good rapport and he often treated me as a confidante, he did not return my phone calls or text messages after he was let go. Liz tried to organize a dinner with Andy in the weeks after Mike fired him, but Andy cancelled at the last minute.

The first time I saw Caryn, a nurse at Rolling Hills, after Andy was fired, she smiled, chuckled, and said, "Well, this is gonna throw a new twist onto your book." A former manager at Rolling Hills, she surmised, "Something must have been wrong with the budget." She echoed the sentiment of others when she said, "I love Andy, but if he wasn't doing his job . . . [trailed off]." Mike hired a new administrator, Regina, less than a month after firing Andy. Regina's style was much more formal, and she set a different tone than the freewheeling and loose culture Andy cultivated. The managers adjusted, slowly. Regina's top priority was reducing agency usage. Regina instructed the new scheduler, Brenda, not to book any agency staff and apparently said that if she told the director of nursing of the "no-agency" policy, Regina would fire Brenda. Regina was hired to improve the budget picture, much like Andy had been hired to improve the nursing home's inspection performance. Regina endeavored to build cost consciousness and efficiency into the structure of the organization, much as Golden Bay had done. Soon after Regina became the administrator, residents complained during the health and safety inspection that there were not enough evening activities. Rather than allocate more funds for activities, as Andy might have done before the budget closed in around him, Regina asked Liz to "volunteer" at the facility every Tuesday night. Although Liz said she felt "burnt out" because a number of her favorite residents died in the previous six months, she agreed to stay late on Tuesday nights.

The way nursing homes are financed ensures compliance with a set of policies that reward practices favorable to cost containment and the enhancement of operational efficiencies. The implications of this system impact the everyday business decisions made at Rolling Hills, Golden Bay, and virtually all other nursing homes across the country. Nonprofits must generate surplus revenue just as much as for-profits. Maggie Mahar put it very well when she used the phrase "No Margin, No Mission" to describe the predicament of nonprofit health services organizations.[13] Institutionalized altruism is unsustainable unless facilities take in more money than they expend. This is made more difficult in light of how altruistic activities are not incorporated into reimbursement or regulatory systems.

The sociologists Paul DiMaggio and Walter Powell wrote what has become a classic article that conceptualizes how organizations, over time, come to look and behave alike.[14] They refer to this process as "institutional isomorphism"—the tendency for organizations to become more similar. Nursing homes depend on the state and must orient their business practices to be consistent with state demands, whether they are for-profit or nonprofit businesses. Medical reimbursement systems reward instrumental acts of care and do not take into account the kinds of community activities that mark the distinctive contributions of nonprofits, generating a system that tilts toward efficient profit taking. Nursing homes, regardless of whether they are investor-owned or nonprofit, must adhere to the same set of policies and are dependent upon the state to remain afloat. Facing fiscal uncertainty, Andy used the same business practices he had learned at the for-profit facilities where he had previously worked. Indeed, these were the tried-and-true techniques of nursing homes against which he now competed, but this time it was too late.

The reimbursement system put pressure on Rolling Hills to prioritize the needs of the needs of Medicare recipients for rehabilitation and discharge at the expense of the elderly poor Medicaid recipients. It forced Rolling Hills to think strategically about revenue, eliciting a move away from their first-come, first-served admissions policy without paying attention to the payer source. However, this does not imply that all nonprofits are doomed. It is conceivable that if Rolling Hills had been a bit more attentive to case mix and established a restorative care program like Golden Bay, they could have avoided the financial crisis that led to the plunge in revenues and eventually Andy's termination. They did not have to game the system like Golden Bay did by extending the length of stay of Medicare residents to be profitable, but they could have done more, without going to extremes, to better manage the case mix and those funds could have been put back into staffing the nursing home.

Rolling Hills' first-come, first-served admissions policy was an important piece of their nonprofit orientation, and it is also a principle that would be good to have throughout the nursing home industry. It is, however, incompatible with the national and state reimbursement policies that provide much higher reimbursements for Medicare than they do for Medicaid. This does not mean that Rolling Hills was necessarily forced to be just like Golden Bay because a nonprofit could be much more strategic in their approach than Rolling Hills. They could have maintained a subset of high reimbursement Medicare and self-pay reimbursements precisely to fund their altruistic activities and to provide high-quality care to poor Medicaid residents. Furthermore, after overextending themselves and getting into financial trouble, Rolling Hills could have gone through a period of reduced altruistic activities until the budget picture was more reasonable and then reengaged in a more careful and sustainable way.

Nursing homes operate within different levels of constraints, from the level of federal and state policy to the level of organizational mission, and they can be relatively aligned or misaligned with each other. Taken together, they have a sizable impact on the experience of work in nursing home care. Rolling Hills ventured, for a time, far afield from what the reimbursement system rewards, and the staff at all levels felt the impact. This question of alignment also has an impact on residents' quality of life, often in ways that are oblique, such as how Medicaid residents were shuffled around the nursing home to make room for Medicare residents. But in other ways the impact is more direct. The next chapter shows how the consequences of the financial crisis at Rolling Hills impacted food and meal service, which is a critical component of quality of life for nursing home residents.

5

Feeding Residents on a Starving Budget

Given the reimbursement system of nursing home care, no nursing home can take a first-come, first-served approach to admissions without jeopardizing revenues. Andy learned this lesson the hard way. He was terminated because of the revenue crisis that developed at Rolling Hills. He ran the nursing home according to principles that were out of sync with what the reimbursement system recognized as care. Although it is hard to ignore that Andy could have managed the budget better, despite his virtues in other areas, the problem he faced is a problem more generally in the nursing home care industry. Residents need placements regardless of their funding source, and a nursing home determined to offer admissions to residents irrespective of their funding source will likely face a revenue crisis. The nursing home industry as a whole remains quite profitable precisely because this is not how most nursing homes do business.

The reimbursement system pays nursing homes for instrumental acts of physical care, providing a powerful motive to have residents more dependent on staff, while implicitly undermining the social and emotional aspects of nursing home care that residents need for a decent quality of life. The regulatory system exacerbates these constraints by normalizing chronic understaffing and work overload. There is simply not enough time for staff to do the tasks they need to perform, let alone the tasks they want to. Reimbursement and regulatory structures constrain nursing homes into prioritizing Medicare residents over Medicaid residents, understaffing over adequate staffing, and instrumental acts of care over social and emotional acts of care.

This chapter continues the analysis begun in the previous one by showing how Andy was forced to cut expenses in the dietary department in an increasingly desperate bid to stabilize Rolling Hills' finances. This budgetary austerity directly harmed residents' quality of life and the morale of Rolling Hills' work force. The entire episode of cutbacks on the dietary budget that I document here was driven by the nursing home's financial crisis. It seems possible that if Rolling Hills had more competent management it could have generated sufficient revenues to fund a more adequate dietary program while continuing with some of its altruistic activities. But the more salient issues are the constraints the reimbursement and regulatory structures impose on nursing home care. Nursing home staff are constrained into cutting corners where they can, and those places are principally in the areas central to the social and emotional well-being of residents. The reimbursement system is not set up to value or reward aspects of resident care that are crucial to residents' quality of life such as meals and activities. At Rolling Hills, meal service became a key area where Andy figured he could cut costs without jeopardizing future revenues, even if it left some residents unsatisfied with the quality of their food.

Much of the research on food in nursing homes has not examined these issues. It has been more narrowly focused on techniques to increase residents' food consumption. Undernutrition is a chronic, often undetected problem in nursing home care.[1] It is also a complex problem caused by a variety of factors, associated with functional impairments such as dementia, stroke, difficulty swallowing, and other medical problems.[2] Psychological problems such as depression, loneliness, and isolation also play a role in undernutrition and are associated with a worse prognosis and higher morbidity and mortality.[3] Intervention studies have found that when the social environment is improved, the food consumption of residents also improves. For example, serving food "family style" in large bowls rather than preplated atop plastic trays, and eating food with staff members together at small tables increases residents' food consumption.[4] A home-like ambiance also helps to increase food consumption and enhance the health and nutritional condition of nursing home residents.[5]

As important as it is to reduce undernutrition, it is also important to increase the pleasure nursing home residents derive from food and meals. Food is about more than the physiological components of nutrition. Meals are an integral aspect of quality of life, especially in nursing homes where it is very difficult for residents to leave and get a good meal elsewhere.[6] Given the long association between care and nourishment, food has a social value that connects residents to a wider social world. Mealtimes allow individuals to relate to other people and to patterns of family life they enjoyed prior to nursing home life.[7] Sitting down for a "family meal" is considered an occasion that demonstrates a commitment to time spent with loved ones,[8] and although nursing home care is far from "home" in any traditional sense of the term, residents want as close of an approximation as possible. They want choices about when, where, and what they eat, food that is comparable in quality and care to a homemade meal, and well-trained staff who care about them and take pride in their work doing the cooking.[9]

The link between food and care runs throughout American culture and is deeply connected to cultural ideals of living the good life. In nursing homes, those connections are weakened as a variety of organizational constraints undermine the experience of pleasure and satisfaction that accompanied meals prior to admission. A qualified dietary staff with the capability to prepare and serve food on time is a necessary component of satisfying and enjoyable meals, yet dietary workers are consistently some of the lowest paid workers in nursing home care and are generally not trained in the dietary needs of the elderly.[10] One scholar argued, "We have delegated one of the most important and challenging nursing care activities to the least educated and lowest paid worker in the nursing home."[11] When nursing homes meet the demands of payment structures and regulatory systems better than they meet the needs of residents, care becomes task-oriented instead of resident-oriented.[12] Floor staff struggle to balance these competing logics that shape and constrain nursing home care.[13] Everyone loses in this system.

"There's Nothin' Nice about the Food"

In the middle of 2007, the year this fieldwork was conducted, state authorities sent a survey to nursing home residents to assess how satisfied they were with their care. Satisfaction was measured along six domains: activities, administrative and personal care staff, food and meals, personal care services, physical environment, and residents' personal rights. Rolling Hills' overall satisfaction score (measured on a 1 to 5 scale, 5 being the most satisfied) was no different from the state average of 4.19 or from Golden Bay's score.[14] In fact, the two nursing homes were very similar across all the domains. Both had lowest scores in the "food and meals" domain, significantly lower than the state average of 3.92.

The state published the above results, but I was provided unpublished results that further broke down Rolling Hills' results. Surveys were mailed to ninety residents or a family member, and sixty-five were returned, which yielded a relatively high 72 percent response rate.[15] Their scores were lowest on ratings of food and meals, with "overall satisfaction with meals" more than a half point lower than the next lowest score. I did not obtain this detailed level of data from Golden Bay, but their similar scores indicate that their services were of similar quality.

Rolling Hills scored significantly lower than the state average on quality, availability, and variety of food. Survey respondents had the opportunity to write open-ended comments about their experiences with the nursing home. The most frequent comments were statements of general satisfaction with the facility; however, among the handful of comments about food and meals, all were negative. One declared, "The meals are looked forward to by residents more than anyone can imagine, the sad part of this is the poor quality of their main meal: mashed potatoes are made from flakes and water—no milk, no butter; *all* vegetables are steamed free of any color, texture or taste; pasta is watery; in general food is tasteless. *No* fresh fruit, *no* fresh vegetables. This is not the military or a prison." Another wrote, "I believe the food should be served to the residents much hotter. I am sure heated dish/containers could be used." A third stated, simply, "The quality of the food needs improvement."

Inside Andy's office was a note on yellow paper. It was taped to the door frame at his eye level. It read, "Complaints provide an opportunity for the nursing home to reevaluate itself and provide better care." Despite this reminder about the value of complaints, Andy did not view the survey results as an opportunity to be seized upon. Given the financial problems Rolling Hills developed over the year, Andy identified the dietary department as a unit to cut costs aggressively. The dietary department was approximately two thousand dollars over budget every month. To clamp down on the budget overrun, he held a series of meetings with Flo, the dietary manager, to insist that she keep food and meals expenses under budget. Flo told me that the budget at Rolling Hills allocated $3.38 per day, per resident for all food and dietary supplies. This is a miniscule amount considering how much nursing homes charge. Moreover, the dietary budget had not increased from the previous year, despite the spike in costs of core foods such as eggs and dairy. Flo claimed her budget was half of what the average nursing home spent on food and supplies. She was embarrassed: "That's why our meals half the time look like shit, because we buy bottom of the line everything. There's nothin' nice about the food. The residents aren't gettin' everything that they should get on a daily basis, and it's just—it's—we can't do it on our budget. Like, it's impossible."

The sad irony of the low food quality is that nursing home residents anticipate meal service perhaps more than anything else, except for family visits. Meals in the main dining room were also the single best opportunity for residents to speak with each other in a way that approximated their social lives prior to entry into the nursing home. Meals were a highly anticipated

opportunity to be sociable amid a daily life that was mind-numbingly bor-
ing. They broke up the daily monotony and offered a chance to interact with
people in a setting that was reminiscent of life prior to entry to the facility.

The main dining room functioned quite a bit like a restaurant; residents
were welcomed and seated, asked what they would like to eat (there was a
choice of drink, two entrée options, and a choice of dessert), and served by
the staff, often managers who rotated meal duties. Managers cleared dishes
from the tables and refilled drinks as if they were waitresses. I often helped
with these tasks. Residents were not allowed into the main dining room
before the official mealtime because there were no staff members available
to watch them and they were not trusted to enter early. Instead, residents
lined up in the hallway just outside the locked doors to the dining room up
to thirty minutes before the doors opened.

Waiting is inversely related to power.[16] It will likely come as no surprise,
then, that residents waited every day to get into the dining room rather
than have staff present for residents to enter at their leisure. Three residents,
Betsy, Eli and Dotty, sat outside the dining room doors each day and waited
patiently to be allowed inside. Betsy, a big woman with white curly hair and a
booming laugh, was accustomed to waiting. She often sat in her wheelchair,
in the activities room, for well over an hour for an activity such as bingo to
start. Her mealtime table mates lived on different units from her, and she
seemed to enjoy the opportunity to be sociable with them, even though
some days they just sat quietly and ate together. Eli rode the elevator down-
stairs every day at eleven thirty, like clockwork. He propelled himself in the
wheelchair and "picked up" Dotty. Dotty was too weak to propel herself several hundred feet to the dining room. Eli wheeled himself behind her, and
pushed her along a few feet at a time, with his one good arm, all the way to
the dining room.

The dining room itself was a large room that seated around forty of the
higher functioning residents at Rolling Hills. Residents who needed more
assistance with eating took their meals in the unit dayrooms, and a few people were fed inside their rooms. The dining room had ten to fifteen square
tables that seated four individuals at each. Name cards were in front of each
seat as staff put residents whom they thought would get along together,
although they could switch seats if they preferred. The room itself had large
windows that overlooked a forest. Wallpaper, homey drapes, framed prints,
and a large fish tank gave the room an ambiance that approached a home,
but the sheer size of the room and the plastic trays of cheap food left no pretense about whether or not this was an institutional cafeteria.

Work-to-Rule

Rolling Hills was the first nursing home Flo had ever worked in, and she confided to me that it would be her last. She was once the chef at a nearby restaurant that achieved the status of a local institution. At that restaurant, she had cooked for many of the residents whom she now cooked for in the nursing home. She said that she loved spending time with the residents and that it was her favorite part of the job, but the budget limitations were a severe source of frustration. From Flo's perspective, "National Nursing Home Week is what set off the whole entire budget problem." The American Health Care Association designates the second week of May as National Nursing Home Week, and Rolling Hills organized daily events to celebrate. The theme was "Treasure Our Elders" and the events were, to my surprise, organized to recognize the staff as much, or even more so, than the residents. Rolling Hills held events each day for a week, the centerpiece of which was an Iron Chef cooking competition. The competition pitted Flo against the chef from a locally owned grocery store, which most staff and residents knew well. Each chef cooked three dishes in one hour using a secret ingredient. Approximately seventy-five residents and staff gathered in the main dining hall to watch the competition, which had the two chefs on opposite sides of a long table filled with food. In terms of entertainment, the event was a smashing success. It also generated good publicity in the local newspaper. But it was pricey. "The Iron Chef cost us $600 alone just in food, and half of it we didn't use, because you don't know what you're gonna use when you do something like that," Flo said. In addition to the Iron Chef competition, Flo made special meals for the staff every day during Nursing Home Week, and treats such as a carnival-style popcorn popper and a cotton candy machine were set up in the front foyer. "It all comes out of my budget," Flo continued. "So Andy knows this ahead of time, and he—I think everybody had a good time at National Nursing Home Week. I think everybody enjoyed everything. But, when the bills came in, it was, 'Why are we?'—National Nursing Home Week cost us three thousand dollars just for that week."

Golden Bay also held events during Nursing Home Week, but they were much more modest. For example, given the "Treasure Our Elders" theme, one day the staff were encouraged to dress as pirates. On another day, they paired residents and staff on a "treasure hunt" around the facility.

Two weeks after the celebrations ended, Andy met with Flo because he did not understand why dietary expenses were so far over the monthly budget. She reminded him of the Nursing Home Week activities and explained the scale of the expenses. Andy informed Flo that at the beginning of the year, she was supposed to build into her budget the costs for special events, holiday meals, and all other functions throughout the year. Flo went back to her office and did the math. "I kinda figured it out and that would like probably make our price per person per meal like one dollar a day," she said. "You know what I mean? It's just not possible. It's not feasible. It can't happen." After that meeting she developed a plan to show Andy, because telling him had not worked, how the food budget was insufficient to meet the residents' dietary needs. She worked with the dietician, who shared Flo's outrage, to begin a novel form of a traditional "work-to-rule" campaign, in which she strictly limited the food and supply orders to stay within the budget for the next two months. Work-to-rule is generally thought of as an action in which workers do no more than the minimum required by the rules of the contract or workplace. Her intent was not to be a good employee and stay within budget; rather, it was to prove to Andy that it was impossible to provide residents with adequate nutrition care within the budget constraints. She said there was no choice but to go over budget in order to properly feed the residents. Flo thought there would be so many complaints from residents, family members, and staff that Andy would have no choice but to agree with Flo and raise her budget to better reflect her department's expenses.

Flo explained, "The last two months, June and July, I was convinced that— 'cause I'm sick of hearing Andy say, 'you're over budget, you're over budget,' so I sat down, I told the dietician. I said, 'Look, the next two months, I'm not gonna be over budget. Let people go complain to Andy that we don't have stuff. Let people complain that we're out of stuff and see what happens, and he'll see what a difference it is.'" She had faith that Andy would see it her way.

Just a few people at Rolling Hills knew that Andy was demanding Flo reign in the food budget. Even fewer knew about Flo's work-to-rule gambit. She did not tell her colleagues about her plan because she wanted them to feel the consequences genuinely and complain to Andy. She had little doubt they would.

I realized that the work-to-rule was being felt by staff when Randi, an activities aide, looked at me and bellowed, "Nobody cares!" We had just escorted about twenty residents, one at a time, down the hallway of the dementia unit to the dayroom. Once there we lined them up around the walls of the small room into a semicircle as polka music played in the background for entertainment. Morning activities were about to begin. Randi planned to serve coffee and snacks, followed by sing-along and then trivia until eleven thirty, when it was time to return residents to prepare for lunch. I was surprised by Randi's outburst because although she occasionally complained about her job, like we all do, I had never heard her so upset about the conditions of work. The accusation that nobody cared was a rhetorical smack in the face to the entire mission of Rolling Hills. I asked Randi, "What do you mean?" As we stood with the waist-high activities cart between us, she pointed down to it and said exasperatedly, "Look at what I have for snacks!" Individually wrapped crackers and cookies were strewn atop the cart, as were bottles of soda, coffee, and large Styrofoam cups. She framed her outrage in the form of a question, "Why can't they get these people something decent to eat?" Then she motioned toward the cups she was about to serve drinks in: "Nobody cares that we have to use these Styrofoam cups! Yesterday I had to serve coffee in those big twenty-four-ounce cups because that was all we had." It was difficult and potentially dangerous for frail individuals with dementia symptoms to handle such large cups filled with coffee. Randi concluded, "Whoever does the ordering does not care!"

The austerity affected not just the snacks provided during activities sessions; it also hit the nursing staff. One afternoon, Stephanie, a nurse, looked up at me over her medication cart and muttered, "This place is going downhill fast." Stephanie rarely cast the facility in a negative light. Her remark, much like Randi's declaration that nobody cared, caught me off guard. Stephanie explained that there was no ice cream for Marilyn. Marilyn was a resident who lived on the dementia unit for just over three years. On the day she arrived, her niece brought her to the facility early in the morning and never came back. It was clear that her family had neglected Marilyn, as she was unkempt on arrival. Now, Marilyn spent a lot of time sleeping or sitting in a wheelchair adjacent to the nursing station. The nursing station is a busy area with a lot of traffic, and Marilyn asked nearly anyone who walked by her, "Miss, where'm I goin'?" The staff were unwaveringly compassionate and tried to soothe her confusion; throughout the day they answered her back, "Right where you are, Marilyn" or "We're going to stay here today."

Twice a day Marilyn ate ice cream that had her meds, ground up, mixed in with it. She, like dozens of residents, had difficulty swallowing, and crushing the pills and putting them in ice cream or yogurt made them easier to swallow.[17] Plus, Marilyn seemed to like ice cream a lot, as it was the only time she quieted and appeared content. If any part of her consciousness felt pleasure, it was when she ate ice cream. Flo's work-to-rule campaign left the facility without those supplies several days every week, until she could afford to place a new order. In the midst of her daily med pass, Stephanie ground up Marilyn's pills to be mixed with ice cream, as usual. Then she walked to the small kitchen on the unit and opened the freezer and found no ice cream. She called dietary and asked them to bring more, but was told that none was left. Stephanie was annoyed at more than the minor inconvenience that Marilyn's meds were mixed with applesauce for a few days. Marilyn may or may not have realized that she was without ice cream, but Stephanie did and it insulted her caring sensibilities. Stephanie wondered aloud how and why the facility could not keep these essential items in stock. I took a chance, and mentioned to Stephanie that the facility could not afford to purchase all the necessary supplies because of the low Medicare census. Her eyes widened and her mouth went agape; it seemed as if she was not sure what I was talking about but she knew that it did not sound good. I was nervous I had said too much, but I gained a valuable insight—she had very little knowledge of how the broader dynamics of the reimbursement system shaped the experience of care work.

Flo explained, "We don't have the proper stuff for med pass, so it's like on a weekly basis, I either hear from Andy complainin' to me in one ear, or I hear the nurses in another ear, like, 'We don't have what we need.'" She continued, "The nurses would call up here, 'How come we don't have this? How come we don't have that?' Because instead of orderin' four cases of yogurt, which we need for a week, I could only afford to get one or two, and it's important stuff, 'cause they need it for med passes and all that stuff." It was not only that nurses may not have had what they needed for dispensing medications; it was that the residents may not have had what they needed for adequate nutrition. Flo said, "Andy wanted us to cut back on dairy products. Well, the residents have to have so much dairy a day. It's impossible. Like, you just can't do it, and we literally, on our delivery days, wait for our milk to come in to serve it 'cause we just don't have any." In fact, one morning in the activities office, Liz, the activities director and a close friend of Flo, told me that she "overruled" Andy upon hearing that the nursing home did not have enough milk for that morning's breakfast. Liz told Flo to go to the nearby supermarket and get some for breakfast service. She said that if Flo was going to get in trouble at work, it should be for doing something good for the residents.

Food shortages were an acute problem, but there were also chronic problems such as the old and broken equipment Flo used to cook. She explained, "We have our regular convectional ovens. We have three of 'em. They don't work [well] at all. We—all our equipment—our grill, half of it works. And this is—we're feedin' more than a hundred people a day and half of our equipment doesn't work and needs to be replaced." The steam table that held food at the right temperature had been replaced because the nursing home was cited by the state for low food temperature during the health and safety inspection. Flo said it was Mike, Andy's boss, who got the steam table replaced. She said that Mike told her, "'If it wasn't for me, you wouldn't have gotten that replaced, 'cause Andy wasn't doin' it.' This is his boss sayin' this stuff to me. I'm like, 'Jesus.'"

They began to run out of basic supplies like cups. A month into the work-to-rule, Flo told the managers that nurses were complaining about serving residents drinks in Styrofoam cups. Randi, the activities aide discussed earlier in this chapter, had complained to Liz about the Styrofoam cups she served coffee in, but residents used them during meals as well. The nurses and Randi all felt serving drinks in Styrofoam cups showed a basic lack of care for residents' dignity. In a managers meeting, Flo explained that the facility needed more "real" cups, but added fretfully that buying them would put her over budget. Perhaps Flo hoped Andy would give in out of shame as the entire management team looked on, and he did. Andy explained, "I know I've been killing you on the budget, but for this you just go ahead and order them and tell me that you're going over budget. We don't serve drinks in Styrofoam cups." Care for residents easily spilled over into care about residents.

Two weeks later, Andy asked the managers, as he routinely did, if anyone had issues or concerns to discuss. Beverly announced matter-of-factly, "We need real plates." She explained that residents ate off paper plates three times a day, and "It's embarrassing to be serving paper plates to visitors." A meal in the main dining room with a resident was a unique opportunity to leave a good impression on a visitor; however, they were serving meals on paper plates and had just begun charging visitors a few dollars for the meal. Again, Andy agreed in the managers meeting to spend more on dietary, and he said that Flo should have done it because "it's a clear customer service issue." Flo was not present for this conversation because she was short-staffed in the kitchen and was preparing for lunch. Serving meals on paper plates diminished the sense of pride staff took in their work, but Beverly also worried that it cast Rolling Hills in a bad light. Aware of the generally terrible reputation nursing homes have in American culture, Beverly was concerned the paper plates and Styrofoam cups contributed to the image of uncaring, profit-hungry institutions.

During this period they also ran out of suitable chairs in the main dining room. The high-back chairs were made of dark wood and had flower-patterned cushions. They were old and tattered and on their last legs. It had been a while since broken chairs had been replaced, and at times there were not enough chairs to seat everyone. When a staff member prepared the dining room for breakfast, lunch, and supper, she often walked to the activities office and took chairs back with her to the dining room. Staff members began to ask each other, "When are we going to get more chairs?" or they declared with righteous indignation, "We don't even have enough chairs!"

Andy said that Mike was coming down on him for budget overruns and that there was no way extra spending would be approved until the next fiscal year.

The last day of July 2007, two months to the day after Flo began the work-to-rule, I happened to be standing in the kitchen when Andy walked in and asked to speak with Flo in her office. He praised her for cutting costs. She intended to stay within her budget but had gone over by about eight hundred dollars. Flo told me, "He came in today and he says, 'You know, you're doing really good on your budget.' He said, 'Last month, for everything, you were over eight hundred,' and he's like, 'that's great.' And I said, 'Yeah, well, have you heard any complaints about anything?' He's like, 'Yeah, I hear it all the time.'" Andy praised Flo, but she felt discouraged. "I'm like, would you rather be over budget, or would you rather have complaints from the residents, the nurses, their family members," she asked me. "We have some people that are on special diets that I can't afford. Like, our—we have gluten-free people. I can't afford to buy gluten-free bread. I can't afford to buy gluten-free pancakes and French toast."

It was several months later that Andy was terminated. Afterward Mike told the managers he had approved a series of repairs and purchases that Andy had not executed. He explained that Andy told him that the repairs were made. Flo seemed to corroborate this charge because she told me that when she informed Mike that there was rust on the floor of the walk-in freezer, he looked at her and explained, "That's been fixed." But it had not. As I stood with Flo in the back hallway near the fire alarm box and the back door, she suggested that Andy lied to the managers and said she was disappointed in him. Minutes later she energetically looked to the future and said that Mike let her order new pots and pans, and that she had priced the cost of new stoves, ovens, and food carts for Mike's approval.

When things at Rolling Hills reached their nadir, managers knew they did not have the financial resources to match other facilities, but claimed they made up for it to the extent that they cared personally about residents. Liz explained, "You might get more effective business-end people than Andy. But you're not gonna get the caring that we do. You know? So what do you want?" One might respond that the choice is not between compassion and nutrition.

Nursing homes are compelled to cut corners in areas that are largely outside of the reimbursement system. Food and meals represent expenses to nursing homes that do not generate revenue. Medical payment systems and the Department of Public Health are not concerned with matters like pleasure and the enjoyment residents get from meals. Medicaid and Medicare reimburse on how much assistance is provided to residents during meals, and regulators care about whether the food is stored and prepared safely. The people who are most affected by low-quality food are the residents, and they have little voice and even less power over their meals.

Scholarship has examined how to improve the food service in nursing homes, with ideas including buffet-style dining,[18] instituting a system for residents to provide feedback about the food quality,[19] and designating a "host" table that selects a favorite meal for the kitchen to make so the host can share a meaningful food memory with other residents.[20] "Flavor enhancement" has also been considered.[21] However, these efforts to improve the food quality are undermined by structural conditions that limit what nursing homes are able to do in the cause of better quality of life. It is all well and good to brainstorm ways to improve food service in nursing homes. Until nursing homes are compelled to improve food and meals through the regulatory system or are rewarded by reimbursement systems for doing so, most nursing homes, particularly those in financial distress, will identify nutrition as something of a money pit with little chance for a return on the investment.

This is about more than just food. Nursing home reimbursement systems have almost completely overlooked the dietary services, activities, and social services departments that are essential to enhancing or undermining residents' quality of life. These departments do not generate revenue and are typically underfunded, understaffed, and simply given far less attention and resources than are needed to create the hospitable, caring communities that residents and their families want. It is not that nursing home administrators and managers do not care about these departments; it is that, as the case of Rolling Hills makes clear, investing resources into areas that do not contribute to revenue streams does not seem like a smart financial move, given the constraints of the contemporary nursing home industry.

Reimbursement and regulatory authorities have overlooked the ways in which mealtimes can enhance the life satisfaction of residents, focusing instead on food temperature and timeliness and ignoring the social and emotional component of a strong dietary program. But what would happen if the dietary services department earned reimbursement money when they involved residents in meal planning, or if there were new regulations that required a certain percentage of revenue to be used for dietary programs and other ways to improve the residents' quality of life? Nursing homes would invest more resources in these departments. The payment structure has got to change if nursing homes are going to give these essential services much-needed attention.

Nursing home care workers have little control over these organizational and institutional sets of constraints. They do the best they can to help the individuals who need their help, but they operate in a context that forces their attention toward reimbursement and regulatory matters. That social context undermines the ability of staff to provide compassionate care to residents. It reduces residents to the embodiment of reimbursable activities and reduces care work to instrumental concerns such as the temperature of food rather than its variety and quality. Given these constraints, nursing home care workers focus on the one thing they seem to have direct control over, the emotional attachments that develop between themselves and residents. They turn, as I will show in the next two chapters, to the symbolic world of emotions to generate meaning and dignity within an institutional structure that seems to undermine both.

6

The Uses of Emotions

Nursing home care workers often felt a sense of frustration and resentment toward the reimbursement and regulatory systems.[1] But beyond how they felt, the actions, interactions, and underlying assumptions that guided their behavior suggested that they were constrained by these systems, nudged into doing care work that seemed to serve the needs of those systems more than the residents. Managers and floor staff faced those pressures and constraints, but given the hierarchical structure of the workplaces, they faced them differently. The managers had to be concerned with the documentation, and those concerns forced them into behaviors like pushing documentation to the brink of the fraud line and putting on a show for inspectors. These were things they did not want to do. The social and emotional care the floor staff gave to residents, when they had the spare few moments in a day to give it, was both essential and nearly invisible. It seemed to many of them that managers cared about money and the state more than they cared about the residents. Normalized and chronic understaffing underlined these challenges, which made it exceedingly difficult for everyone to do the tasks that had to be done without cutting corners here and there, whether it was a nursing assistant who skipped a resident's scheduled shower to catch up on the morning rush or a manager who filled out documentation and then asked a nursing assistant to sign it.

This structure undermined what staff members throughout the work hierarchy in both nursing homes said they valued most, caring for people who needed their help. Given this context, workers drew from a reservoir of memorable moments and experiences of doing care, which seemed to them outside the scope of the reimbursement and regulatory systems, to construct a sense of meaning and dignity in their work. Sociologists have shown how workers struggle with organizational contexts that devalue their work, yet still manage to construct their jobs, and their selves, as dignified.[2] People engage in interpretive processes to endure and even enjoy certain elements of work that are by most conventional standards not enjoyable. In this chapter and in the next chapter, I use data from both nursing homes to make arguments about how staff used emotional and rhetorical strategies to construct their work in a positive light. Workers used a wide range of interpretive frames to form meaningful connections with certain residents. Workers at all levels of the hierarchy at both nursing homes told stories, recalling tales of emotional closeness that, they explained, were perhaps the most valuable and rewarding part of the job. These emotional and rhetorical strategies sought to give their work positive meaning in a social context that is fraught with things to feel bad about. Emotional labor was a skill, learned through the trial and error that comes from experience, that helped staff construct dignity at work. Yet emotional labor did more than that. It was also a resource to exact compliance from residents. The more experienced staff were more skilled at emotional labor and applied emotions in certain situations to get residents to behave how they wanted. The less skilled workers, often relatively new nursing assistants, were less successful at using emotional labor to induce compliance from residents. In these moments when emotions failed the staff, residents seemed to control how care unfolded, often with negative consequences for all parties.

Managing Emotions

When Ted, a lifelong New Englander and an avid Red Sox fan, passed away at Rolling Hills, it was important to his wife June that the staff remember him. In the last few weeks of his life, Ted's mental acuity declined rapidly and a quiet, gentle man easily became confused, frustrated, and angry. June brought a framed five-by-seven black-and-white photo of Ted smiling in his wheelchair to the unit. The photo was a reminder, for the staff as much as for June, of the "real" Ted prior to his descent into dementia. Maria was Ted's daytime nursing assistant, and she was touched by June's gesture. Just before Ted died, Maria spoke with June. I asked what she said, and Maria explained, "I thanked her for letting me take care of him." June donated Ted's Red Sox–themed clothing protector to Eli, the man Ted shared a table with during meals in the dining room. In addition to the framed photograph and the clothing protector, June brought a stack of thank-you cards for the unit's nursing assistants. Inside of each card was a wallet-sized photograph of Ted and a five-dollar gift card to Dunkin' Donuts. Although the staff members graciously accepted the gift, it was a violation of a long-standing policy that prohibited gift exchanges between staff and residents or residents' family members.

A few days later, the managers required the floor staff to sign a document that acknowledged their awareness that gifts were prohibited. This was not a coincidence; it was a clear and direct response to June's appreciative gesture. The management at Rolling Hills and Golden Bay had established modest policies to mitigate favoritism; the most prominent was the ban on gifts between staff and residents or their families. This policy was difficult to enforce, since a gift in exchange for better care could be given in a private area without the knowledge of managers. It did, however, establish a formalized set of organizational boundaries on emotions. Ted's nurses, Stephanie and Caryn, accepted the reasoning behind the policy for living residents, but thought it was wrong to prohibit gifts from families after a resident had died.

Gifts that had monetary value were not permissible, but gifts that had symbolic value were accepted and often proudly displayed. Behind the desk of the nursing station of the dementia unit was a tattered card, held in place by a piece of scotch tape. The card was from the family of a man who had recently died. It read, "You are all angels of mercy" and thanked "all the staff for your compassion and kindness with John. Especially thanks for whoever got his pillow and brought it to him in the hospital. He was holding it when he passed. We will never forget this. Thank you." Another card I found on Liz's desk in the activities room at Rolling Hills read simply, "Thank you very much for being such a good friend to our mother, Paula. We were honored to have you at her funeral. God Bless." Stacey, a nurse at Golden Bay, kept an angel made of hand-blown glass in her car. The first resident she became emotionally attached to gave it to her. "It was a long time ago, like eight years ago," Stacey explained. The resident knew she was dying; multiple organs were failing. Stacey worked the overnight shift, and the resident was often awake all night long. "We spent a lot of time just hanging out and talking. She died, but you know what? Before she died she handed out little blown glass angels to all of her favorite people. I got first pick, and I still have it, it's in my car."

Thank-you cards, flower arrangements, mementos, and photos from family members of residents who had recently died often lingered on the units for weeks. This in itself is a form of impression management, in that the nursing station is a stage to display the close ties between staff and residents and their families. In addition, these items materially codified gratitude in a way that did not violate the gift policy.

Organizational policies such as the gift ban marked the boundaries between staff and residents. Although staff and residents formed meaningful attachments, certain boundaries were very rarely crossed. For example, most staff members had one or two favorite residents, and some small shows of favoritism between that staff member and "her resident" were said to be an inevitable part of the job, but it would have been extremely unusual for anyone to invite that person home for dinner. Cynthia said it was beneficial for staff to think of residents as fictive kin, "like family," but Golden Bay did not set organizational conditions that would cultivate such relationships. Another manager worried about emotions blurring the boundary between staff and resident. She explained her reasoning: "Sometimes that line—they may talk to them like they're talking to a family member, perhaps. And you know, they're residents. It's kind of hard to describe. You know? Like [in a parental, annoyed tone of voice] *you were up, walking around your room again. You know you're not supposed to.* You know? It's got, I guess, a little scolding tone. And I know they don't mean any harm by it, but you kind of have to remind them sometimes, you know you're still the nurse, and they're the resident. And this is their home. And you need to treat them respectfully." Heather was concerned that emotional connections undermine the staff's professionalism toward residents and could lead to unfair harshness toward the more rebellious residents.

Aside from organizational policies, informal rules, and managers' attitudes, there was an institutional context that exerted control over emotional labor. This context was exemplified by the reimbursement and regulatory agencies' concern for instrumental acts of physical care and the implicit devaluation of care for residents' social and emotional needs. It was worsened by the normalization of understaffing. There were simply not enough resources to provide the full spectrum of care that nursing home care work required. This tension epitomized institutional care more generally.[3]

Given the structural constraints of the workplaces, staff turned to the symbolic world of emotions to give their work positive value. Emotion work, a concept developed by Arlie Hochschild, refers to the process of aligning our inner emotion and our outer displays of emotion with the normative expectations of how we are supposed to feel and act in a given situation.[4] When emotion work is done for a wage, it is referred to as emotional labor. Workers can perform emotional labor on a continuum, with total sincerity at one end and total cynicism at the other. Staff in the nursing homes often spoke with complete sincerity about the emotional attachments they felt toward certain residents. In fact, workers explained that they became emotionally invested in residents' care for a number of reasons, often related to a common trait. Insofar as these affinities are based on similarities, they are deeply social. The staff and residents tended to be demographically similar white women, even though separated by age and perhaps social class. Yet the attachments are deeply asocial in that they exist outside of, and perhaps prior to, social interaction.[5] Below I describe some of those attachments. I chose them because they provide some sense of the variation in how emotional attachments formed, but I could have just as easily chosen other examples. The "realness" of the emotions between staff and residents is not the issue that I am primarily concerned with. Rather, I endeavor to show that the emotional labor component of care work—aligning privately held emotions with the publicly valued and normative emotional context of the workplace—was useful as a skill that helped staff manage the demands of their work.

Daphne and Ronald

Sometimes staff and residents became emotionally attached because they shared a similar life-defining experience. For example, Daphne, a nursing assistant at Rolling Hills discussed earlier, recalled clearly the first time she felt connected to a resident. "That was back in 1996. That was very emotional," she said. Daphne was one of the first nursing assistants to open her work world to me. She was a white woman in her early forties with long, straight blonde hair pulled back into a ponytail, a single mother of young children. Within weeks after I started doing fieldwork, we began to chat, and before long we talked freely, often while I assisted as she made beds or passed out trays of food to residents.

Daphne and Ronald, the resident, shared a similar life-defining event: both were estranged from their biological families, except for one sibling with whom they each remained close. "So that really hit home," Daphne said, "and I really knew where they were coming from, so I just kind of formed that bond with them." Both went through the experience of being ostracized from their family, and as a result Daphne was easily able to relate with Donald, but especially with his sister. Daphne told me,

> The day he died his sister just totally broke down and she said, "What am I going to do without you?" She said [to her brother], "you can't leave me. I have nobody else. You're the only one that I have. You're the only family that I had. I have nobody now." And it was like something you would see on a TV show, it was so dramatic. And I just stayed in there with her, you know, and *I felt like it was me* in that situation, and what if my brother had died, where would I be left? And I remember coming out and crying and crying and crying in the linen closet.

Daphne was upset because she cared about him. But she cried for more than that; she had connected with Ronald's life story in a personal and intimate way. She could not help but reflect on her own life and how the two were similar. She also empathized with Ronald's sister, and imagined how she would feel if it was her own brother who had died. Daphne said that grief over a death does not become easier to manage with time, but rather depends on unique relationships with residents.

Frankie and Maude

Shared life experiences were one of the ways that staff and residents connected emotionally. Staff members explained other ways, such as a shared religious denomination. Frankie, a nursing assistant on the rehabilitation unit at Golden Bay, had a particularly close relationship with Maude and her family based on their Catholicism. Frankie was a young man who was tall and strong, enabling him to care for the bigger residents whom the smaller women had difficulty maneuvering. Although his coworkers liked Frankie personally, they also complained that he worked too slowly. Frankie said his work pace was intentionally slow because he encouraged residents to do as much as possible independently, which he viewed as an important element of rehabilitation. Residents appreciated the extra time, he explained.

Frankie had a special relationship with Maude that, in his mind, was the result of divine intervention. Maude had terminal cancer, Frankie said, "and my heart went out to her 'cause she was such—just one of the nicest ladies here." She was close to death: Frankie thought Maude had only weeks left. A devout Catholic, he went to church after his shift ended, something he did often. His priest instructed all the parishioners in attendance to give someone a rose. Frankie decided to bring Maude a rose: "You know, I just had this feeling that I should do this," he explained. Frankie bought a rose, went to Golden Bay, but realized there were no adequate vases. He left and purchased a vase, and when he returned Maude's family was in her room. "They asked me," Frankie said, "why did you bring this rose? It's very, very nice. We asked St. Teresa to send my mother a rose." Frankie replied, "Well, it's a funny thing, 'cause I had a feeling I should bring her this rose."

"Very pious woman, very pious," he described Maude, "and she had a special devotion to St. Teresa." Her family told Frankie, "You know, we were praying in church today and we said, 'would you send us a rose, so that we know that you're gonna take care of mom?'" The family asked God to send their mother a rose, and hours later Frankie showed up with one. After Maude died, her family sent Frankie a special gift to remember Maude by, "and I keep that and I treasure that. It's not the thank-you card. It was the funeral card, with the prayer on the back. And she's in my prayers." Maude and Frankie's common faith led to a relationship that transcended the traditional resident-caregiver boundary. Maude's family acknowledged that with the funeral card they sent to Frankie. Frankie said, "If they had given me a basket or something, I'd be like 'oh, that's nice,' but the funeral card meant a whole lot more, and for that reason I'm going to carry it awhile, at least in my heart I'm going to carry it with me for the rest of my life."

It was Frankie's coworker, Kirsten, the rehabilitation coordinator, who explained that "reimbursement comes from the heart." This remark suggests only a slightly veiled criticism of profit-driven care and represents an effort to find a source of meaning in care that transcends monetary concerns. The reimbursement she referred to is the inner satisfaction that comes from caring for individuals who cannot care for themselves. The primary reward for caring about residents, in addition to caring for them, was the gratification that came from feeling that their job has a sense of purpose greater than their paycheck affords. For Frankie, it meant a lot that Maude's family validated the authenticity of their connection.

Cindy and Edith

When I asked Cindy to tell me about a resident she became emotionally connected to, the first thing she was, "If I do I'll start crying, 'cause what stays in my head is Edith, you know, 'cause she broke my heart." Then she chuckled and explained, "You know, Edith used to be a pain in the ass. It's funny 'cause the ones that you really don't like at first, that are like a pain in the ass, they're the ones that you end up getting really attached to. It's amazing." When Edith came to Rolling Hills she expected to stay a few weeks for rehabilitation and return home; but she never regained enough strength. Confined to a wheelchair, Edith became a long-term care resident on the bustling rehabilitation unit. At first her room was located next to the nursing station, but it was so noisy she could not sleep. Her room change request was granted, and she moved to the first room on the unit near the main hallway. It was still a high-traffic area, but Edith enjoyed sitting in the doorway, quietly humming or chatting with visitors as they walked by. The unit manager said Edith was "good public relations"; she was a relatively healthy resident who sat in her doorway and could make an uncomfortable visitor feel less anxious about nursing homes. Edith's new room was on Cindy's assignment. When she first met Edith, Cindy thought to herself, "'Oh my God, how am I going to put up with her?' Cause she was kind of obstinate about doing anything. She'd drive me nuts, and then I turned out loving her so much."

Everyone knew Cindy and Edith had a special connection. Their relationship included neither heart-to-heart talks about life and death nor private conversations about the intimate details of their lives, yet the relationship was close in a way that was uniquely their own. They enjoyed inside jokes nobody else understood, and at times they seemed to have their own secret language. When Cindy worked sixteen-hour double shifts, Edith let Cindy nap in her bed while on break. They shared a bracelet: one day Edith wore it and Cindy wore it the next. In the mornings, Cindy woke up Edith to the tune of Frank Sinatra's "On the Sunny Side of the Street." She explained, "This is no lie, Jason—it would say, 'Come on to the sunny side of the street' and then it would go, 'Start walking, boy' and I'd go 'Start walking, girl.' I mean I'd sing it to her every morning. Every morning." Cindy said, "I did crazy things with her. I loved her so much. We had so much fun." Sometimes Edith sat in the activities room playing cards with her son. Edith hated animals, and occasionally Cindy would sneak up from behind Edith while she played cards, crawl down on her hands and knees, and start barking like a dog. It was a playful relationship.

I was with Cindy when she found out that Edith died. We were at a staff member's wedding reception; I approached Cindy to say hello, and she immediately told me that Edith was not well. Cindy had stayed with Edith after her shift the night before ended to tend to her bedside. A staff member who overheard our conversation tapped Cindy on the shoulder and rather casually informed her, "Oh, she died last night." Cindy burst into tears and sobbed uncontrollably while her colleagues hugged and consoled her. She cried out, "She was my friend!" and "I can't believe nobody called me!" A few weeks after Edith died, her daughters stopped by the facility to thank the staff personally for their care, and to drop off a basket of Yoo-hoo drinks for staff and residents on the rehabilitation unit. The Yoo-hoos were an inside joke: when Edith sat in the doorway to her room, wearing her signature hat with her head bowed, she would whisper "yoo-hoo!" as strangers passed by. Edith's daughters looked for Cindy, but she was at a nearby restaurant on her lunch break. Edith's daughters found Cindy at the bar. Cindy explained,

Edith used to wear this little blue—my favorite color is blue, and she'd tell me hers was too, I think 'cause it was mine. And her daughter came and I go, "That's my bracelet" and she goes, "It's Edith's." I go, "It was mine too." I mean it just, I started crying, so I'm like, "Oh my God" because we'd share that bracelet; one day she'd wear it, the next day I'd wear it. And she [Edith's daughter] took it off her wrist and gave it to me. And then she gave me an envelope and she goes, "We just want to thank you so much for giving mom all the care." And it just broke my heart, you know. And then I opened it, and they gave me a hundred-dollar bill. So I mean it really, it meant a lot. It wasn't the money thing, but it meant a lot for me that they came to find me.

While the cash bonus made an impression on Cindy, there was far more value and impact to the interaction itself. It validated the sincerity of Cindy's emotional labor. These are a few examples of the intensity and authenticity of emotional labor, but there are others. A nurse at Golden Bay explained, "They become like family. They really do, and they see you every day, forty hours a week or more. You just connect with them." Stephanie, a nurse at Rolling Hills, said, "My closest ones, I have to say is Faith and Edie. I love Faith. Oh, I love her to pieces. I really do. I have to probably say those are my closest ones, you know. I love them guys to pieces. I mean I care for them all very much but those two I just love to pieces." Although these relationships may be "like family," they are definitely different from family ties. It's uncommon for someone to say they love their family "to pieces." Perhaps this is a different kind of love, a different kind of emotional rhetoric from familial love.[6] But in all of these cases, workers expressed a deeply felt connection with residents.

Beverly and Sally

Emotional labor did not always produce these warm and fuzzy feelings. Sometimes emotions were so intensely felt that staff members fought with coworkers and supervisors about the care of a resident. For example, Beverly, who was a manager by the time I met her but had spent many years as a nurse on the floor of a large nursing home, told me a tale about the time she risked her job because she gave a dying resident her last wish. As I sat in her office on a snowy winter afternoon, I asked about how her career had developed and she explained, "One time I almost got fired from County Nursing Home." County Nursing Home, a state-run facility, was six floors high and held hundreds of beds. It closed in the 1980s, and many of the staff members moved to newer private nursing homes such as Rolling Hills and Golden Bay. One of Beverly's residents, Sally, was in her fifties, relatively young compared to most nursing home residents. She had metastatic lung cancer. "She said to me, 'Bev I'm dying. I'm dying because I smoked cigarettes. I got lung cancer. I might not be here tomorrow. I want a cigarette.'"

Beverly had told this story many times over the years. As the story went, she explained to Sally that a cigarette would make her sicker, but Sally insisted, "That's what I want. I want a smoke." Beverly marshaled the aides on the unit and had them move Sally—lying in her bed—to the dining room. "I gave her a smoke," Beverly said. "I got a cigarette and lighter, and I stayed right with her, and she smoked. She only did it once. She only wanted one. She didn't even smoke the whole thing." Although Sally worried that Beverly would be fired, Beverly told her, defiantly, "Well, so be it." Sally died a week later and Beverly "got called to the office because, of course the CNAs told on me." Beverly told her boss, "If you need to fire me, you need to fire me. That was that patient's last dying wish to have a smoke." She declared that Sally was cognitively competent and was lucid enough to make an informed decision. Beverly added that what she did was the same as handing a diabetic a hot fudge sundae, and as she told the story to me, it was as if she still making her case: "It was her last wish," she explained.

More than twenty years later, Beverly still has the letter Sally wrote to her before she died. "It says that she wants me to remember always that I gave a dying person what they wanted," Beverly explained, "that I made her life, you know, better by that moment because that's what she wanted, and that she felt people need to do and say what they need to do at the end of their life and that I should never forget that I did that for her, no matter what." Beverly never forgot. This story is her moral compass that directs her attitudes toward care for the aged. Do whatever necessary to give a dying woman her last wish, even if it puts your job security at risk. In telling this story, Beverly established herself as a caregiver who cared more about her resident than she did herself. When I mentioned the story to Liz, she said, "I'm happy Bev told you that story" because to her it symbolized the selflessness and giving nature of nursing home care work.

Rebecca and Faith

Rebecca explained that the first time she met Faith, "She came in with her daughter and they sat down next to me and I took her hand and held her hand, and it was like an instant bond. We just connected. Faith just really felt comfortable; she would talk to me and laugh and hug my arm." Faith's dementia intensified slowly. Her behavior patterns worsened after a brief hospitalization. Whereas Faith once had a healthy appetite and a calm, warm demeanor, she now became easily distracted and irritable and barely touched her breakfast. Standard morning procedures required Faith be woken up and ready for breakfast by eight thirty. Rebecca said that waking her at that hour, "It was just totally frustrating Faith, making her agitated, where she would get combative. She wasn't as strong first thing in the morning like she was before she went into the hospital."

Rebecca told Stephanie about the difficulty Faith had eating in the morning. Rebecca suggested feeding Faith breakfast in bed because the activity in the dayroom distracted her. Stephanie agreed, but only days later other nursing assistants on the unit objected. They said it was unfair to allow Rebecca to stay in Faith's room for the duration of breakfast while they passed all the other trays, helped residents eat breakfast, and cleaned up the trays. "So it was making them work a little harder and it took a little longer, and it was annoying them and stressing them out and frustrating them," Rebecca admitted. Bonnie argued to the unit manager that taking Rebecca off the floor to feed Faith breakfast put everyone else behind schedule. Rebecca said indignantly, "Well, in my opinion it's not what's best for us; it's what's best for the residents. I mean, I thought they had rights!" She said her coworkers thought only of themselves, meanwhile: "I used to leave every day just totally burnt out and frustrated and felt like crap because they don't deal with Faith every day, they don't know how she is, except for when she comes out in the dining room and she's screaming and yelling. I'm the one that takes care of her every day. I know how she acts; I know how it makes her feel." The unit manager scheduled a staff meeting to discuss the issue. Rebecca explained in that meeting how it was better to feed Faith apart from the other residents. It relaxed her, she ate more, and she had begun to gain weight. The unit manager agreed, but weeks later changed her mind and required that Faith be fed in the dayroom. Reluctantly, Rebecca agreed because "I didn't want to get written up. That was my fear, always getting written up or getting fired because I'm not doing what my boss tells me to do." "I dragged her out of bed every morning," Rebecca explained that it made Faith angry, upset, and confused. She ate less and lost weight. "She was left to fend for herself," Rebecca said with an ache in her voice. To alleviate staffing pressure, the unit manager fed Faith in the dayroom. Rebecca said, "You know, I'm not trying to brag, but I knew what worked for her to get her to eat, but she [unit manager] didn't know her little tricks and ways to get her to eat." When Rebecca explained her "tricks" to get Faith to eat, such as bringing in some food for herself to sit and eat quietly with her, "they would just look at me like I was strange." The understaffing at the nursing home clearly made a difference here, because if there was adequate staffing, then all the residents would be able to eat in the place and time that was best for their health and well-being, rather than at the place and time that was best for the nursing home schedule.

Rebecca continued to work, but was not earning enough money to support her family. She began to work overnight shifts for the hourly wage differential, but found it was too stressful and tiring to do that while raising children. Plus, "Faith was breaking my heart," she explained. It did not take long for her to receive a better job offer from a nearby hospital for substantially more pay. She asked Rolling Hills to match the pay, but they could not. Rebecca resigned:

> REBECCA: And that was the most difficult thing I've ever done.
> JASON: Why?
> REBECCA: Because being there for so many years you build bonds with the residents. You form really close attachments. Even though they tell you in the nursing field you can't form attachments, you can't help it; you're only human. So it was very hard on my last day. I couldn't even go in and say good-bye to Faith because it would've just been too hard for me emotionally. So I gave her a hug and a kiss the day before. And then I think the last day, when I got her back into bed, I gave her a kiss and I just had to leave. I just left the room, you know, gave report, and I left the floor. So that was really, really hard.

Rebecca's emotional labor did not generate feelings of meaningful fulfillment as much as it bore sadness and grief. She felt guilty about leaving Faith behind for reasons that included higher pay and a better schedule. Perhaps, in my interview with her, she wanted to emphasize how much she cared about Faith so that she could present herself as having made an honorably difficult decision. But she also felt strongly enough about Faith to engage in a protracted battle with her supervisor and coworkers about her care.

Constructing Dignity, Inducing Compliance

I expected that since the staff were around illness, disease, and death, they would use some kind of "detached concern" or "affective neutrality" to make sense of nursing home care work.[7] Yet what I found was far from detachment or neutrality. I found genuine concern. Given a workplace structure centered on the particulars of documentation, reimbursement, and regulatory compliance, staff took full advantage of their emotional attachments to residents. The staff used emotional labor as a resource to construct dignity, with varying success, but they also used it to induce compliance among residents, also with varying success. Emotional labor is partly about inducing certain emotions in customers, whether it is the feeling of safety or comfort or reassurance, all of which were emotions staff wanted residents to feel. The staff members who could induce those states, while also taking satisfaction in themselves, were the most skilled at utilizing emotional labor, and those skills were more common among the experienced staff.

Consider Bonnie, a nursing assistant at Rolling Hills for nearly twenty years. At first I was surprised when she explained to me, "I like the feisty ones, the ones that put up a fight." It is not a coincidence that a nursing assistant who likes challenging residents would stay on the job for so many years, as care workers who do not think like Bonnie would eventually find work elsewhere. She empathized with new residents in their adjustment from home to a much more confined living space, and said, "You just took away all their freedom." Bonnie further explained, "When you get through the spunk and the fight in them and they trust you and they cooperate with you, it's like you have done something amazing. You have helped this person adjust to a life that they have no choice but to adjust to, and it's really rewarding to see them adjust. You know what I mean? It's very fulfilling."

Bonnie did not think of her emotional labor as a means of social control; however, residents' behaviors are manipulated through such connections. This is the skillful use of emotional labor: what could produce emotional dissonance instead produced pride and fulfillment for herself while at the same time she induced the feeling of comfort in residents who had difficulty adjusting to a life of institutional care.

For many care workers, the most rewarding residents were shy, aloof, or even hostile and noncompliant with their medication regimen or dietary restrictions. They posed a challenge for staff, and when staff members were able to break through and establish trust with a resident, they viewed it as an accomplishment. Emotional labor as a form of "heroic caring" gave them meaning and dignified their work. I found this pattern of talking about the emotional components of nursing home care in both nursing homes, among both the floor staff and the managers.

Louise was a nurse at Golden Bay. She explained that her favorite part of working on the long-term care unit was that she got to know the residents, many of whom for years before they died. Like Bonnie, she explained that she liked the "really difficult and grumpy residents" because she is often the one to crack their ornery shell. "You just have to learn their ways, butter them up, make them laugh," she said. "I have residents that will refuse their pills for thirty days and then you just have to make them laugh and BS with them and they learn to trust you, and then they start doing what they're supposed to." Louise enjoyed this challenge. It was emotionally gratifying, yet at the same time she used the attachments with residents to manage their behavior. Randi, the activities assistant discussed previously, also explained that the most rewarding residents were not necessarily the friendliest or most cooperative individuals. "The amazing thing is a lot of the ones that end up being your favorite are not the nicest people and they're not the sweetest people. They're just interesting, you know?" she explained. "I can remember one lady, that, oh my heaven, she could be a real witch, but we just loved her." Randi said that the nice and friendly residents already got a lot of attention and she preferred to concentrate her efforts on the less outgoing individuals who sometimes required extra attention. Like Louise, Randi noted that these individuals pose a welcome challenge: "If you're persistent enough, they'll let you in." This is essential work that takes skill and determination—and it is completely invisible to nursing home reimbursement systems.

Laura was a nursing assistant with over ten years of work experience in nursing homes. She told me a story that demonstrated how the most experienced and skilled nursing home staff used emotional labor in a way that made them feel good while also inducing compliance in residents. Laura reminded Dorothy, a resident with dementia, of her estranged daughter, "and she was very happy I was back," Laura told me. She explained, "She called me her daughter, and out of respect I called her mother. It made her feel good." Laura wondered aloud if there was a "boundary issue" when she allowed Dorothy to refer to her by her daughter's name, but surmised that even if it was problematic, it was worth it because she ate and slept better, was more relaxed and generally better off because she believed her daughter was there with her. Dorothy was physically and verbally aggressive with staff members when they provided direct care, a work hazard that is more common than people realize.[8] Laura said, "When I was there I was able to bring her back, and everyone thought that was wonderful that I was able to pull her back." Emotional attachments were a tool Laura mobilized to control unwanted behavior. Dorothy's health improved because of Laura. When Laura returned from a weekend off, she found her "mother" had a severe stroke. "I was feeding her every meal. I worked my shift. I went home. I fed my kids. I came back and fed her supper. That's how close we were." A few weeks later she died, and although Laura had accepted death as a part of her job, it was still emotionally difficult for her: "But everybody made me feel good that I did a really good job with her. And it was difficult, but she was happy. She was happy. She felt like she had her daughter back, and I gave that to her and I was very pleased to be able to do so. And I'll never forget that. I'll never forget it." The sense of being "like family" was how Laura helped to control Dorothy's aggressive behavior, but it was also part of how she constructed a sense of doing meaningful work.

Beverly's story along these lines was perhaps most compelling. She was the admissions coordinator at Rolling Hills, and her entire career had been in nursing home care. She told me one of her earliest and most memorable stories about the emotions embedded in care work, which, she explained, "has driven me all these years to be in long-term care." She described her previous workplace, County Nursing Home, back in the early 1980s: "It was sort of like a warehouse type thing," and she said it was six floors high and housed hundreds of elderly sick individuals. She underscored that this was prior to the Nursing Home Reform Act of 1987, when physical and chemical restraints were often used to control individuals with dementia. "It wasn't like it is now, with all the documentation and ombudsman and all of that," she said. Beverly cared for severely debilitated individuals; most of them were unable to get out of bed and did not speak due to advanced Parkinson's disease or dementia. Although the residents could not talk, Beverly said, "You know, there was just a spot in my heart and I would always say, 'good morning, how are you?' and blah blah blah. They never talked to me. You know, they couldn't."

Undeterred, Beverly made one-sided small talk. A nursing assistant overheard her in a resident's room: "This little CNA came and she said, 'why in the heck are you talking to her?' and I said, 'I'm talking to her because she's a person and some place, some level, I believe that every one of these people is there. Not on our level, but some level. It might be just a smile, but they're there.' I said, 'that's why I'm here, because I want them to know they are cared for.'"

Beverly developed a strong affection for Patty, a resident who did not speak. Beverly's colleagues thought Patty was mean because she pinched them when they tried to assist her. She also refused medications. Beverly said she thought the pinches were a way to communicate: "So, instead of thinking that she's mean," Beverly explained, "maybe you need to look at whether or not that person is really in there." As months passed by, Beverly chatted to Patty, who did not appear to respond. "I'd do the same thing every day," she said. "The CNAs thought I was kind of weird, but I'd go in and I might sing, or I'd make small talk, just do my own thing with them."

Finally, all the attention paid off, and Beverly had a moment she would never forget, one that crystallized the reasons why she loved being a nurse. She was in Patty's room, "I was kind of teasing her a little bit." Then she asked Patty to open her eyes, and to her amazement, "she opened her eyes and smiled at me." What was initially a delightful surprise became a routine occurrence, as every morning Patty opened her eyes, smiled at Beverly, opened her mouth, and took her medications. The way Beverly told the story, this experience became a lesson in care work that she taught her colleagues. She brought the nursing assistant who said she was "weird" for talking to the residents and had her watch as Beverly provided care to Patty. Patty opened her eyes, smiled, and took her meds without hesitation. "And I said, 'and that, right there, is what this is about. So if you're having a lot of trouble with these people, you need to change how you're acting with them, because they're there.'" Beverly's moral tale peaked when the nursing assistant who doubted her admitted to having learned her lesson: "One day she comes up to me and she said, 'You know Bev, you're right, I can give Patty her meds now, because I'm talking to her, but the other girls they can't.'"

There is no way to know how much of Bev's tale is accurate, particularly since the event happened so long ago, but its accuracy is not as important as how it works for her as a lesson in caring. That she made a point to tell me the story in such detail is itself evidence of how it frames her understanding of what people who do nursing home care work should be doing. She explained that staff members, if persistent enough with emotional labor, could induce compliance in even the most difficult resident, and that this brings great joy to care work. But I do not wish to imply that everyone walked around happy and dignified all the time; certainly they did not. As Clifford Geertz explained, "Nothing has done more to discredit cultural analysis than the construction of impeccable depictions of formal order in whose actual existence nobody can quite believe."[9] Sometimes emotional labor failed and interactions broke down into unresolved conflict.

When Emotions Fail

The more experienced staff members were particularly skilled at marshaling emotions to induce compliance among residents while also generating feelings of pride and dignity at work. Staff members learned these skills through informal processes of trial and error, learning from veteran staff members and generally spending more time on the job. The newer, less experienced staff members were not as able to deploy emotions in a way that brought about the rewards of their skillful use. One example that shows the difficulty less experienced staff members have in using emotions happened in my presence when I watched staff members prepare Betsy, a resident at Rolling Hills, to take a trip to her doctor's office. Andy described Betsy as a "tweener" because her severe dementia and schizophrenic symptoms required care that oscillated between what nursing homes and psychiatric facilities provide. Although she maintained residence at Rolling Hills, she had spent several weeklong stints at a nearby psychiatric facility when her behavioral symptoms worsened. She regularly intruded into other residents' personal space, hoarded food and other items, and needed "one-on-one" monitoring for months, in which a nursing assistant was required to follow her continuously throughout the unit and document her activity every fifteen minutes. Tall and broad shouldered, Betsy ambled up and down the hallway, arms held behind her back, her head slightly bowed and tilted to the left. She spoke quietly to herself, about herself, in a third-person voice.

Betsy's nurse, Caryn, asked Amy, a newly certified nursing assistant, to get Betsy in a wheelchair, which would then be strapped into the paramedic's van waiting to take her to the doctor's office. Amy put the wheelchair in front of Betsy, who was seated in a high-back chair across the hall from the nursing station. Betsy became visibly anxious, her eyes widened, and she gripped the chair's armrests. Her legs rocked back and forth. First, Amy took a friendly approach and kindly asked Betsy, "Can you please get in the wheelchair for me?" but Betsy said she did not want to do that. Amy asked again, her tone this time an octave higher to sound even friendlier, "Honey, could you please get in the wheelchair so we can go to the doctor?" She gently touched Betsy's upper arm to coax her along, but Betsy, who was at least fifty pounds heavier than the short and thin Amy, resisted easily. Amy decided to seek help from more experienced staff members. Stephanie and Bonnie cajoled Betsy into the wheelchair without much trouble. They "helped" Betsy into the wheelchair with a standard "two-assist" technique: each staff member reached underneath Betsy's shoulder, between her arm and chest, hooked her arm inside theirs and pulled her up, slowly turned her toward the wheelchair, and then set Betsy down. While Amy asked Betsy to get in the chair, Stephanie and Bonnie told her and then moved her.

Mere seconds after Betsy sat in the wheelchair, the paramedic who drove the van wrapped skillfully a seatbelt around Betsy and turned it so she could not unsnap it. It was clear he had done that many times before. Stephanie explained to Betsy that she needed to visit the doctor, but that seemed to make her more nervous. Frightened, she muttered rhythmically, "She hates wheelchairs" and "She doesn't want to go," talking to herself about herself. Amy tried to bargain with her. She told Betsy she would be coming right back, but Betsy, having spent a week recently at a psychiatric facility, did not believe her. Then she asked if Betsy wanted ice cream for the ride, but she did not. Nor did she want coffee. Seemingly out of options, Amy called upon even more emotionally potent rhetoric. She calmly kneeled down beside her, rubbed her hand up and down Betsy's arm, and said "I love you" as sincerely as she could. Betsy had nothing of it: "Well I don't love you! I hate you!" she said. As a new nursing assistant,

Amy looked upset and unsure what to do. She repeated, "I love you," but it did not work any better the second time. Betsy spoke aloud, repeatedly and rhythmically, "She's scared. She's scared. She's scared." At this point Betsy's nurse, Caryn, resorted to indirect force. Caryn took control of the situation and pushed Betsy's wheelchair down the hallway. Betsy put her feet firmly on the floor, which made it very difficult for Caryn to push the chair. Caryn deftly spun the wheelchair around and pulled it down the hallway backward. Betsy put her feet down again, but this time they dragged as Caryn led her off the unit and out the front door.

Amy's emotional labor did not induce the calm state in Betsy that she had hoped it would. The perceived authenticity of emotional labor was important for controlling unwanted behavior of residents. Betsy seemed to see through Amy's inexperienced use of emotional labor, knowing that Amy didn't really love her and that it was a transparent attempt at manipulation. In most interactions with service workers, authenticity does not really matter that much. We are not truly concerned about whether, to use Hochschild's famous example, a flight attendant's pleasant demeanor is authentic or an act.[10] But given the intimate character of nursing home care work, the perception of authenticity matters more. The staff learned to use emotional rhetoric as a skill, not from management above, as Hochschild argued, but from an experiential and informal process.

Take the experience of Rita, for instance. Like Amy, Rita was a recently certified nursing assistant. After only two months of working at Rolling Hills, her assignment called for her to shower Faith, a woman with severe dementia and confined to a wheelchair. Faith, a retired teacher, was heavy enough that she needed to be transferred using a Hoyer, a crane-like contraption that lifted residents up in a mesh basket to move them from wheelchair to bed and back. Rita and Marlene, a seasoned nursing assistant, wheeled Faith from the dayroom to her bedroom to prepare her for the shower. I accompanied them. Faith became visibly nervous as they brought the Hoyer lift to the edge of the bed and began to strap her in. Her eyes moved from side to side and she held her arms out flat on the bed. As the lift began to take her into the air, she asked anxiously, "Where are we going?" Marlene told her, lightheartedly, "We're going for a ride" as Faith, who hung in a mesh basket suspended about four feet high in the air, was repositioned to be lowered over the shower chair, which looked like a toilet seat with arm rests held up by stool legs. Rita tried to assure her, "Faith, we're going to make you smell like roses." Then Rita wheeled Faith into the bathroom, under the showerhead, and closed the door. I stood in Faith's bedroom and listened to Rita and Faith struggle in the shower. With the soft gushing sound of water falling from the shower, Faith alternated among confusion, anger, and fright. Rita tried to give quiet emotional comfort, not only to Faith, but also to herself:

FAITH: I'm gonna kill you!
RITA: I love you.
FAITH: You're terrible!
RITA: I'm not. I'm washing you up.
FAITH: You stop it—right now!
RITA: Faith.
FAITH: I don't care what you said!
RITA: I'm gonna make you smell like roses.
FAITH: Owwwww.
RITA: Behave.
FAITH: Leave me alone! Leave me alone! Don't do that! I'm dying!
RITA: No you're not.
FAITH: Get away from there!
RITA: Faith, I'm cleaning you up.
FAITH: Get away! [moaning several times] Get away! They're coming after
   you! Now get the hell out of here! I mean it!
RITA: Faith.
FAITH: Get out of here now! Oh my god, what are you doing! You are a
   stupid moron!
RITA: I'm a stupid moron, huh?
FAITH: You're gonna see me! Get away! Get away! Get away!
RITA: Faith, I am not hurting you.
FAITH: I am not hurting you yet, but when I do it's gonna be unbelievable!
RITA: I'm washing your bum. It's dirty. [water stops]
FAITH: Oh, thank god! I got to get a hold of these people! You do not do this,
   you understand!
RITA: I ain't mean to you, I love you. I'm gonna tell you the truth, I love you.
FAITH: I'm dying!
RITA: No, I won't let you, I love you too much [kiss sound].
FAITH: Look what you did!
RITA: I put your shirt on you.
FAITH: I can't take anymore! I can't take anymore! You are a dumbbell!
RITA: Why thank you.
FAITH: Oh god! This has been the worst, worst, worst thing I have seen ever
   in my life! Are you satisfied?
RITA: I love you too, Faith [in an exasperated tone].
FAITH: What?

RITA: I love you too.

FAITH: Yeah, sure [in a sarcastic tone].

After the water was turned off, Rita opened the bathroom door and looked at me. Then she quickly turned and opened the room door, peered in the hallway, and asked for help. Then she wheeled Faith, still seated in the shower chair, into the bedroom. Rita and Faith both looked scared. Rita held up her hand and showed it to me; it trembled with anxiety. "She hit me sixteen times in the head," Rita explained. Her colleagues were not surprised to hear that Faith was physically aggressive. Marie said she could be "brutal" and that "she knows where it hurts." After Rita struggled to get Faith dressed and ready to sit in the dayroom until lunch, she walked out of the room and quietly muttered to me, "I just want to finish my assignments and get the fuck out of here."

Emotions were most likely to be perceived as insincere or otherwise insufficient in cases like Amy's and Rita's—when inexperienced staff members used emotions in a transparent way to help them perform especially sensitive acts of care work. The staff received little, if any, training about appropriate emotions in the workplace.[11] Rather, they learned from experience. Sometimes staff spoke to each other about techniques to handle difficult residents. The more experienced nursing home care workers were generally more successful at using emotional labor to induce an emotional state in residents, such as calm and the feeling of being loved. It was the new staff who had not yet learned how to deploy emotions effectively.

A recent study of nursing lamented the "nearly complete absence of attention to emotion work in official time allocations and staffing criteria."[12] The intensification of work in nursing homes has increased demands to do more work with less support, leaving less time for vital social and emotional support for residents.[13] The floor staff's work routines consisted of a particular set of assigned tasks that must be completed within a given amount of time, and they were held accountable to these expectations. This in itself impeded the floor staff's ability to establish and nurture relationships with the residents, which required intent and substantial time on the part of individual staff members. Yet my analysis also points to the power of emotional attachments, an essential piece of nursing home care work. While management and the larger structure of nursing home care imposed tasks and limits on floor staff in an attempt to control them, workers used emotional labor to push back. Even managers who had little direct contact with residents, such as Beverly, recalled emotional attachments made years earlier when they worked on the floors. Others fondly remembered residents now gone. These attachments, and memories of attachments made, dignify paid care work.

The staff by and large did not view their workplaces as sad or depressing, even though it had its moments. Instead, they said they were grateful for the emotional attachments with residents and they welcomed opportunities to make residents' last days a bit happier, brighter, and more comfortable. Staff who continued to work in nursing homes, rather than leave the field, had developed rhetorical strategies and self-conceptions that moved beyond the obvious sadness of working with individuals who get sick and die much more often than they get well and go home. Take the finding that some staff members identified with "difficult" residents. Residents who "resisted" care were in some ways the most recognizable images of fully able individuals who have not succumbed to illness, disease, or the obedience that life in institutional care exacts. Perhaps staff imagined that if they were the residents, they would be "difficult" too.

Consistent with the overall experience of care work, there was more variation within the nursing homes than there was between them, suggesting a model of emotions that is more flexible than Hochschild's formulation allowed.[14] To apply Hochschild's model in a straightforward way to Rolling Hills and Golden Bay, Golden Bay would likely put greater emphasis on teaching workers to manipulate patients' emotions because it was a for-profit home and emotion is a key dimension in which nursing homes compete—but that did not happen. I expected floor staff to perform a version of emotional labor broadly consistent with Hochschild's model and that managers, especially at Golden Bay, would more or less instruct workers how to "properly" emote, especially given the low autonomy over work conditions that nursing assistants have over their work. I also expected variation between the two nursing homes—that the nonprofit would be more caring than the for-profit. I was ready to believe this, but that is not what I found. Emotions were more self-directed and did not simply reproduce organizational goals. Staff had emotional attachments to residents, but not because of organizational imposition, direction, or even encouragement.

Hochschild's central finding that emotional labor happens has been validated time and time again, which has led some to describe the legacy of *The Managed Heart* as "pervasive but shallow."[15] Although that is true in a sense, it elides some real advances and new directions in how sociologists make sense of emotions on the job. One line of research inspired by Hochschild's work concerns the extent to which managers can truly control workers' emotions. For example, service workers can come to view their highly routinized scripts as a source of power, even as a kind of rhetorical shield against insults from irate customers.[16] Emotional labor "does not have uniformly negative consequences for workers," especially when workers are provided with some autonomy on the job.[17] Expanding on this theme, emotional labor among supermarket checkout clerks has been shown to be self-directed, not driven by management, and to lead to a sense of personal fulfillment when workers create friendly relationships with certain customers.[18] Waitresses have been known to use emotional labor to their own ends, manipulating customers into giving bigger tips.[19] Indeed, workers appear to have much more control over the production and deployment of emotions than Hochschild's formulation had originally allowed.

Sociologist Randy Hodson has argued, "Workers from all walks of life struggle to achieve dignity and to gain some measure of meaning and self-realization at work."[20] The care workers I got to know were strategic actors who extended autonomy to construct dignity. Thus, in crafting a caring self,[21] floor staff positioned themselves as superior to managers along a symbolic hierarchy of emotional attachments. This was a means of constructing dignity at work.

I did not seek to understand the world residents lived in so much as the world staff worked in, and as such I never sought the consent of residents to interview or collect data about them. Nevertheless, given the relational character of emotions, it is reasonable to speculate that emotions worked similarly for residents as they did for staff.[22] Life in institutional care is one of daily and repeated indignities and entails a loss of freedom that many people fear they will experience when they reach old age. Emotional ties to staff can become an anchor for residents as a crucial source of dignity. For most residents, family visits are few and far between. While very few residents used the kind of family ideology that was prevalent among staff, it was obvious that so many residents genuinely appreciated and valued chatting with staff members. The staff, in most cases, were their tightest attachment to a wider world beyond institutional care. Although staff members rarely revealed personal information about themselves, and usually did not have the free time to do so, they still took time to engage in routine social pleasantries that residents appeared to enjoy.

While it is likely that these attachments often generated dignity among residents, it is not difficult to imagine that some residents used emotions to manipulate staff to do what they wanted. One resident, for example, admitted to a staff member that she faked crying to get the staff's attention. Another occasionally received flowers from a manager with whom she shared a close relationship. A third resident routinely threatened to call the Department of Public Health if his requests were not granted. In all these cases, residents more or less explicitly used emotions to get the staff to do things they wanted. Overall this is a more nuanced view of what emotions do than Hochschild's model implies. Where Hochschild emphasizes the production of emotions for organizational purposes in a way that is neatly tied together, what I found was a bit more lawless. Emotions are not so easily managed. They are sometimes out of control as well as in control or used for control. They can serve organizational purposes, but they can also be turned against the organization. Emotions are a contested terrain and are—at times—unmanageable from the point of the nursing home managers. But they are also sometimes unmanageable from the point of view of the workers themselves.

7

Making Sense of Death and Abuse at Work

"I had a resident, Priscilla, who everyone thought was very precious," Heather explained.[1] Priscilla was on death's doorstep and had suffered for years with the symptoms of advanced dementia. Priscilla's advance directives were not on file, a common problem among the elderly at the end of life.[2] Faced with wrenching end-of-life decisions, her children fought bitterly over how to proceed. Heather dealt often with these issues, although not quite as complex as this particular case. She held individual meetings with the adult children and stressed the need to focus on "what would your mom want?" Eventually one of the children produced a set of advance directives Priscilla had signed before dementia took control of her mind. Heather made copies for everyone, and had a group meeting with the children, some of whom had flown across the country to see their mother one last time. After each met with Heather, they held a separate family meeting and agreed to carry out their mother's wishes. On the very night that Priscilla's family came to an agreement and stopped fighting over her care, she stopped breathing. Heather explained, "It's like she felt, 'my family has come together. And now they're at peace, and they're letting me go.'" Heather spoke with the family after she died, "I said, 'You know I just feel like your mom sensed that you guys were all okay with each other, and that maybe she was detecting some animosity amongst you. And now she was okay with it, so she could just let herself go.'"

Heather's tale exemplifies a type of narrative I heard over and over again: staff said that nursing home residents had control over the timing and circumstances of their death. Yet they also said that residents were powerless to control their aggressive outbursts. The selective attributions of intent by staff members positioned residents sympathetically and created for the staff a situated moral order in which dedicated staff provided compassionate care to sympathetic, deserving residents. These two sets of ascriptions are counterpoints because both involve understandings of intent that are ultimately unknowable and do not hinge on whether or not individuals actually choose when to die or whether to strike the staff. Staff attributions of intent reflected their emotional needs.

Human agency—the notion that individuals have the capacity to act independently and to make their own choices, relates to a central issue in the social sciences: how individuals act meaningfully, with intent and with the feeling of freedom, yet nonetheless reproduce what looks very much like social structure, something that persists over time and appears to have its own organization and logic. Viewing agency as a cultural object rather than a state of being, as I do in this chapter, pushes our understanding of the power and limits of the concept beyond current debates, which have had the tendency toward the reification of agency as an object. Agency is not a *thing* that individuals may or may not possess; it is, in practice, a set of understandings, ascribed to a set of behaviors, deployed to create the meaning of interactions and behaviors. The issue of whether people have agency is not germane to how and under what conditions people use a rhetoric of agency, as a conceptual resource, to describe, classify, and understand social activity.

Jaber Gubrium's classic ethnography *Living and Dying at Murray Manor* analyzed the social organization of care in a nursing home, and described how the institutional culture, and the emotional culture that supported it, constructed residents as "waiting to die." Staff implied that residents had no choice but to wait for God to take them. On the other hand, staff physically restrained and chemically sedated violent residents, suggesting their belief that those individuals knew what they were doing. Those attributions of agency differ from those I observed; but the differences are no contradiction. Attributions of intent are historically situated, and in the years since *Murray Manor* was published, the professional philosophies, staff trainings, and regulatory frameworks of long-term care have all changed significantly.[3] These collaborative forces shape how agency is ascribed and denied.

Attributions of agency are put to work in ways that maintain social norms. In a fascinating case study, researchers examined how a family attributed "competence" to their child, whom medical experts judged to be severely mentally impaired.[4] The family, convinced their child pretended to be impaired in public, used rhetorical techniques to reinforce their belief in the child's full competence. A similar point was made in an analysis of how participants in twelve-step groups made attributions of agency.[5] Participants explained other participants' behavior with the selective use of agency. Normative behavior was attributed to the willful actions of individuals and deviant behavior was attributed to mental illness. A concept of agency even more deeply situated in interaction than George Herbert Mead's is evident in caregivers' attributions of "hidden minds" to patients with advanced dementia.[6] This chapter builds on this scholarship by examining how staff used a rhetoric of agency in novel, creative ways, and as a practical resource to interpret behavior within a set of constraints shaped by workplaces.

People make attributions of intent about others' motives in a way that helps them make sense of behavior.[7] For example, Hochschild showed flight attendants were trained to imagine rude passengers as scared and childlike, unable to control themselves.[8] In this way, staff redirected blame away from passengers to preserve the notion that they were worthy of assistance. In a set of observations closer to my agenda in this chapter, a study of boundary work in nursing homes argued that staff did not think of slaps, pinches, and punches from residents as "violent" to preserve the traditional boundaries between care givers and care receivers.[9] The staff at Golden Bay and Rolling Hills asserted that residents could not control their aggressive outbursts, but their attributions extended further than the evidence supported. The staff invoked a rhetoric of agency spontaneously to assign or assuage others' responsibility for behavior. In doing so, the staff managed the emotional stress of nursing home care work and recast agency as a moral concept.

"Everyone Has Their Own Schedule": Ascribed Agency

As I hung up my jacket in the activities office at Rolling Hills, Liz informed me that Mabel was "catching the bus." Euphemisms aside, she meant that Mabel was dying. She asked if I wanted to see Mabel, and I skittishly accepted her offer. We walked down the hall to the locked dementia unit, and as I said hello to Stephanie, Liz waved me into Mabel's room, where she stood in the doorway. The lighting was low and Mabel's bed was against the wall. Her nightstand was under the window by her left shoulder. She was covered to her neck in blankets with a homemade blue crocheted throw on top. Mabel lay motionless, pale and yellow, with her mouth agape as if she was frozen in mid-yawn. She was breathing just five times every minute, each inhalation punctuated with a surprising snort and gurgle. Her lungs were filling with fluid, and she had what nurses call the "death rattle," the sound produced by a dying individual as saliva accumulates in her throat, having lost the reflex to swallow. I stood behind Liz as we quietly watched her. Soft music played in the background, and two morphine-spiked lollipops rested on the bedside table. Our eyes were hypnotically fixed on Mabel. "She probably won't close her mouth again," Liz explained. "There are all these stages to dying." A few quiet moments passed, and before we left the room Liz straightened Mabel's blanket. A few hours later, she was dead. To me, Mabel appeared helpless. But this is not how Liz or other staff members thought of death. In their eyes, Mabel was not helpless. Far from it.

Both nursing homes organizationally embraced the concept of "active dying." Patricia, the staff development coordinator at Golden Bay, described active dying as a set of physiological changes in the body that point toward the end of life, such as decreased eating and fluid intake, changes in breathing patterns, and mottling of the skin, particularly in the feet. She added that when someone is actively dying, he or she is in some sense aware the end is near. This was a standard definition of active dying in palliative care, but in practice it took on a far more general and taken-for-granted meaning among nursing home care workers. I asked Patricia if active dying meant the resident had only a matter of hours or days left, and she explained, "Well everyone has their own schedule," and that the active dying process could take days or months.

Rolling Hills encouraged nurses to continue their education and distributed articles to them about common issues with which staff in nursing homes have to contend. One of these articles was titled "The Last Hours of Living: Practical Advice for Clinicians." It described the typical signs and symptoms that indicate active dying and offered advice to clinicians for how best to prepare loved ones for the death of a family member. "While we do not know what unconscious patients can actually hear," the report states, "at times their awareness may be greater than their ability to respond. It is prudent to presume that the unconscious patient hears everything. *Advise families and professional caregivers to talk to the patient as if he or she were conscious.*"[10] It suggested that staff and families should give the patient permission to die because the person may feel not allowed to die.

In the eyes of the nurses and nursing assistants, dying residents were known to "hold on" until the family arrives or "let go" just after the nurse left the room. They shared many stories of this genre with me. Stephanie, the nurse discussed earlier, explained, "I've noticed the residents don't want to die with a family member in the room. I don't think I've had one resident die with a family member in the room, not one. And I've only had one resident who died with the CNA in the room. They always—and I mean literally thirty seconds after you walk out of that room—they go." One morning on the Rolling Hills' dementia unit, Stephanie was the charge nurse for Peg, a resident who was actively dying. Peg's lungs were filling with fluid. Staff refocused their efforts, instead of working from a framework of "curative care," they moved to "comfort care" measures in which medical interventions are intended not to prolong life, but to make death comfortable and dignified. Stephanie was in Peg's room with a few nursing assistants when Peg stopped breathing. As they waited for Peg's heart to stop she suddenly, and surprisingly, regained her breath. After this episode, she explained, "You know, it's—they—a lot of them *like* to go alone." Stephanie added, "It must be something so personal and intimate. They need to be alone to do it, to go." In her view, Peg was aware that she was being watched and mustered the strength to regain breathing because she preferred to die alone.

Joanne, the director of nursing at Rolling Hills, also told me stories about residents who chose to die. When I expressed skepticism, she stated firmly, "Oh, it's a true thing. I've seen women hold on until that last child comes from three states away to get there to say good-bye." Lucy agreed, "I see it all the time. I think you see it more with women than I do with men; where they just wait to see all of their children before they—it's like they get this last burst of energy or fortitude or just so they can have the opportunity to say good-bye. I'm not sure what it is. But yeah, I have seen it."

Angelina, a nursing assistant at Rolling Hills, described a similar burst of energy among the actively dying residents. She told me about a resident who had severe multiple sclerosis. Having stopped eating and drinking water, she was dying. Then, "she had this burst of energy and she wanted to get dressed," Angelina explained, so she dressed her in nice clothes and sat her in a chair, rather than the bed she had been in. Her family came in, "They walked in, they walked out, and they said to me, 'Do you see what I see?' and I says, 'Yes, surprise!'" Angelina was happy she got to dress the resident in "pretty, pretty clothes" and pleasantly surprised the family. The resident died just a few days later.

Ariel, a nurse at Golden Bay, had worked in nursing home care for twenty years and had many stories to tell. She described a dying woman whose family was coming from far away to see her one last time. "So we were doing— literally hour-and-a-half updates. We told her her family was coming and she said, 'Oh, I'm so happy—I'm so happy that they'll be so happy to have seen me,' past tense—past tense, 'to have seen me.' That was a little odd. You pick up on little things like that." The family arrived to see their mother in the dimly lit room. Music was playing, as it often is when residents are actively dying. Ariel said, "Literally, the family walked into the room. They said 'hello,' and ten minutes later, she was gone."

Ariel theorized that elderly people hold on and wait for family because they understand the significance of closure. Young people, she said, do not want their family to see them sick and prefer death. As supporting evidence, she told me a story of a young boy she cared for who was dying of cerebral palsy. The boy's family was on vacation when he got most ill. Against the wishes of the boy, Ariel contacted the family to inform them of his deteriorating condition, and his parents rushed home immediately. Ariel explained, "He said, 'Well, I don't want my mother to cry' and literally three hours later, before they got there—gone, just gone. And he knew. I mean, he knew. He clearly knew. He had made peace with it, you know."

Stacey told me an amazing story along these lines. She explained that twenty years ago in another state she was a nurse at a facility that housed geriatric, psychiatric, and mentally retarded populations: "just cram 'em all together" she joked sarcastically. One of her patients was a Baptist preacher who was nearly killed by a massive stroke. Before the stroke he was a gregarious and talkative guy, but once stabilized after the stroke, his speech was severely impaired—all he could do was count from one to ten and say "fuck." "He would just sit there," she explained, "four, three, two, one fuck! six, seven, eight, nine fuck!" His wife came to visit, "and I'll never forget this," Stacey paused dramatically. "She turned to me and yelled 'I can't do this anymore! That's *not* the man I married!' and left the facility in tears. Less than an hour later he was dead." There was no doubt in Stacey's mind that the events were much more than a mere coincidence. This story, repeated so long after the events occurred, serves as something of a cautionary tale, told not because it is representative but because it is extraordinary. Stacey staked out a position in which her residents control when and how they die that operates beyond anything she can do to save them.

It was easier for staff to ascribe agency when it seemed like a resident had lived a long, full life only to quietly slip into a deep sleep and never wake up. Toward the end of my fieldwork, for example, a resident passed away a few days after her 103rd birthday. The proverbial "cute old lady," Heidi could not talk but was alert and oriented to her surroundings. She was known for holding up her hand and raising her pointer finger, pinkie, and thumb in the "I love you" sign to staff and visitors. After she died, Victoria admired, "she was continent until the end." Marlene spontaneously told me she felt Heidi was waiting until her 103rd birthday to pass away, and when I asked why, she simply said, "Because she could. Maybe it was her goal to live that long." Crystal agreed, "People wait for an event, graduation, birth of a baby, yeah. I don't think it's coincidental."

Active dying, the rhetoric of agency, is robust enough to accommodate a number of circumstances. Yet these attributions of intent are largely unsupported by any evidence that dying people can actually control the conditions and timing of their deaths.[11] The firm belief that residents have power over death helped the staff to manage the emotions that come with caring for individuals who will die under their care.

But the rhetoric of agency was not so robust that it fit all circumstances—in fact, sometimes the logic broke down. People died under circumstances that made it difficult or impossible to claim plausibly that death was a chosen act. Edith's untimely death was one such circumstance; this well-liked, basically healthy elderly woman died shortly after an untimely accident. Edith was the resident discussed in the previous chapter who had a uniquely strong relationship with her primary nursing assistant, Cindy. She often sat in the doorway of her room and sang or hummed quietly as the hours passed. It seemed like everybody knew her, and people often stopped to chat for a few minutes. One Saturday afternoon as she sat in the doorway, a dietary aide pushed a heavy food truck that was filled with forty lunch trays down the hallway and accidentally rolled it over her foot. Edith went to the emergency room. Less than a week later she had a stroke. Less than two months later she was dead.

The facility developed a counternarrative to explain what had happened. They said that new medications, not the trauma of the accident, caused Edith's stroke. This may have helped them in terms of legal liability, but it did not help them mitigate the emotional weight of the accident. Edith's death had many of the same characteristics staff used to ascribe agency, but no one dared to say she had chosen the circumstances of her death—quite the opposite. The sadness and grief focused on a woman whose health rapidly declined and who died after an accident; they were not focused on a woman who had chosen the timing and conditions of how her life would end.

This counterexample illustrates what staff achieved when they spoke of death as a chosen act. The rhetoric of agency made death palatable. The most emotionally troubling deaths in the nursing homes were those that could not be conceptualized as an act of agency on the part of the dying. It is of course inevitable that residents will die; everybody on staff knew that. One way staff managed the emotional intensity of caring for people who would die in their care was by thinking of it as a powerful act of final choice. This framework is consistent with the "revivalist discourse" of death that emerged from the palliative care movement and emphasizes the role of dying as an opportunity for personal growth.[12] Attribution of agency also neutralized organizational failure. Cynthia told me that she actively tries to counter the idea that nursing homes are a "death sentence." She wanted people to think of Golden Bay as a place where people come to live, not die. Liz said much the same thing. When I began my fieldwork she explained, "This is a place where people come to *live*." The organizational goals were to foster an emotional climate of dignified living; the rhetoric of agency neutralized the fact that most people who walk into a nursing home do not walk out. Finally, attributions of agency dignify death in a total institution such as a nursing home. Its residents have been stripped of dignity in most conventional senses. They have often spent their life savings on nursing home care, have sold or lost their house and have very few possessions, have lost their physical capabilities, mental capabilities, or both, and endure a pernicious loss of privacy. Much as in "total institutions,"[13] residents are told when and what to eat, when to shower, and where to sit, and they often spend hours at a time simply sitting in their wheelchairs, not doing anything. Those deemed at risk of falling wear alarms that erupt when the residents stand or move too far on their own. They have almost no control over the circumstances of their lives, and one way staff can give residents some semblance of dignity is to say they have control over the timing and condition of their deaths, their very last act of life.

"That's the Alzheimer's Talking": Denied Agency

Much to my surprise, physical abuse was an everyday occurrence in both nursing homes I visited. Most of it occurred on the dementia unit while staff assisted residents with personal care in bathrooms and the unit's shower stalls. I had assumed that any aggressive outbursts would be directed at residents from frustrated, impatient, and poorly trained staff. But I quickly learned it was the other way around.[14] A recent study of workplace assaults against nursing home care workers by residents found that 59 percent of certified nursing assistants had experienced an assault with major soreness, cuts, bleeding, or bruising within the previous twelve months.[15] Violence among individuals with symptoms of dementia is a complicated phenomenon that may occur for various reasons including environmental stress, unmet resident needs, cognitive decline, and a history of violence prior to disease onset, yet nursing home management and staff largely accept, tolerate, and expect violence against care workers.[16] This was true of both Rolling Hills and Golden Bay. While the management and the Department of Public Health rigorously investigated allegations of abuse by the staff, verbal and physical violence toward the staff was a routine occurrence and not treated as a problem to be aggressively managed. The staff denied that residents intended to be aggressive, a claim that rested on neither more nor less evidence than the ascription of agency around death. In both cases, the key point was not the presence or absence of human agency, but the ongoing creation of a set of understandings with which to interpret behavior.

Both nursing homes maintained an organizational silence about violence in the workplace. In fact, the leadership of both seemed unconcerned with workplace violence until it was so disruptive that it altered staffing patterns due to workplace injuries. This happened at Rolling Hills, where about a half dozen staff members were injured while performing care on Bud, a big, imposing man who was recovering from a hip fracture. The injuries prompted Joanne to organize an educational seminar titled "The Basics of Alzheimer's Disease" led by a social worker from the local Alzheimer's Association. This effort focused on retraining staff on how to approach residents with advanced dementia with a comforting tone of voice and unmistakable body language. In the first fifteen minutes of the three-hour presentation, the trainer from the Alzheimer's Association asked the assembled staff members to raise their hands if they had been hit by a resident, and all of them had. She said, "You may feel like they know what they are doing," and Maria whispered "No, that's not it" loud enough so everyone could hear. The managers could have focused on retraining staff members to provide person-centered care in the shower or to allow certain residents to be given a towel bath, both of which have been shown to dramatically reduce aggression toward staff members, but instead they relied on the same training material they provided to staff the previous year.[17] The trainer displayed an overhead slide of two brains scans that had become familiar to Maria; she had been through this training before. One of the images showed a normal brain, the other showed a brain deteriorated, particularly in the frontal lobe. The trainer asked, "So, if someone with Alzheimer's hits you, are you going to get mad?" "No," Maria said, with a chuckle. For emphasis, the trainer said, "This is the image I keep in my head all the time. It reminds me of who the caregiver is, and who the care receiver is."

Maria told me a story that showed just how dangerous work in nursing homes can be for nursing assistants. She was working an overnight shift and heard commotion coming out of a room down the hallway from the nurses' station. A resident was in a rage and throwing things around the room. "It was my job to go in and make sure his roommate was safe," she explained. He threw the leg rest to his wheelchair through a window, shattering it. "He's lunging at us, grabbing at us, it was very scary." Maria called the police. "I mean it's a scary situation. It's a very scary situation because you don't know what to do. And sometimes it's hard to deal with. But then you go to the classes and you see that they have no control over those emotions, over how angry they are. Or how they're responding to things. It's just—it's part of their dementia." Maria had cared for individuals with dementia for years and explained that she had "grown to love their explosive outbursts." Rita, a recently certified nursing assistant who struggled to assist Faith in the shower, was not so accustomed. Yet she did not fault Faith, who apparently struck Rita whenever they were in the shower together. I interviewed

Rita only days before she was fired for working too slowly and asking for too much help. I asked her about that shower, and Rita explained, "I took a deep breath, counted to ten, remained calm, and just it's, granted I was a little shaky on the inside, but other than that I knew if I didn't have patience or give her the reassurance that she was okay, and why we're washing up then I wasn't going to accomplish anything." Caryn, who was working that day, explained, "They don't understand they have feces all over them and they need to be cleaned up, so they hit."

Daphne told me she used to get hit or cursed at every day on the job. I asked her what that was like, and she explained, "It can get difficult because physically it's harder on us because we're getting beat on. So you're fighting with this person in the shower, hoping that they don't jump out of the chair and slip onto the floor, or in the process you're getting soaked because they're grabbing the showerhead and they're drenching you because they're so angry. So it's heartbreaking, just because inside you feel frustrated, but then feel so guilty because it's not their fault. You know, they just don't understand." Daphne described work conditions that could make even the most empathic care worker angry—not angry with the residents, but angry with the management who did nothing to protect them. Because aggressive residents could not control themselves, managers were absolved of any responsibility for mitigating the potential for violence against staff.

I asked Louise, who had worked in long-term care for decades, for a story about a challenging resident, and she told me one that was "the worst I ever had":

> He was probably about six-three. Climbed out of his bed, grabbed my wrist or my shoulders and was pushing me against the windowsill. And I was like leaning really hard against the window. My butt on the windowsill. And he was just pushing. Trying to push me out the window. And he was a strong guy. I don't know what the heck saved me but that was probably about eight years ago. Other staff saw him and pulled him off me. But that was the scariest thing that's ever happened to me. And a lot of it is they can't understand that they're doing it. So that's what you have to understand. The resident probably doesn't know that they're doing that. That took me a long time to realize.

While Louise and others had come, over time, to think of residents who had violent outbursts as unable to control themselves, Marlene viewed the outbursts as positive expressions of emotion. She said, "When a resident is attacking you, they're venting their aggravation the only way they know how, and for them I think it's physically better to vent than hold it in. So, if you walk by a resident and they just punch you or something, you know, they feel better even though they really didn't mean to hurt you sometimes. You know you've done something for them."

Occasionally the idea that residents were powerless over their aggressive impulses broke down. One such case involved Bud; he hit staff members as they tried to assist him, and the staff were convinced his actions were intentional even though they also believed that he had advanced dementia. Bud was a physically imposing man who was admitted to a room on Bonnie's assignment. He was rehabilitating a fractured hip but was put on the dementia unit because of his symptoms.[18] Although Bonnie at one point told me that she liked caring for the "feisty" residents who "put up a fight," Bud was not someone who Bonnie seemed to enjoy caring for. Bonnie said that Bud was sexually inappropriate with her and that other nursing assistants egged him on as if it was funny. "He will be grabbing my breasts, grabbing my crotch, and they will be laughing and joking, 'Oh, he wants to kiss you!'" she explained. Her colleagues' reactions angered her, but she was also angry that Bud laughed after he abused her. His laughter was Bonnie's evidence that he knew what he was doing. This attribution of intent—that Bud intended to harm Bonnie—infuriated her.

The gendered character of the interactions played a significant role in the emotional repertoires and strategies staff used to connect with residents. Emotional attachments came out of a foundation of their shared experience as white women, often mothers, growing up in the same area at roughly the same time. With the nearly all-female workforce, there were no male nursing assistants available to care for Bud and protect the women staff members. There was also a structure that took for granted the physical, verbal, or sexual aggression nursing assistants endured as a daily aspect of their work. Given the history of institutional abuses in long-term care settings, managers spent a lot of their time maintaining regulatory compliance. This monitoring contributes to the well-being of nursing home residents, especially with aggressive investigations of allegations of staff members' "rough handling" of residents. But regulatory monitoring does not protect workers from potentially dangerous residents. Instead of having workplace protections from aggressive residents, nursing home care workers, in most cases but not in Bud's, did rhetorical backflips to suggest that aggressive residents were acting without intent—that they did not in fact know they were being aggressive.

Evenings on the dementia unit were particularly hectic because many residents went through "sundowning," a phenomenon in which dementia symptoms increase in the late afternoon and early evening. I observed one evening as two nurses and four nursing assistants struggled to care for forty residents, dozens of whom seemed to have an exacerbation of their dementia. The staff served and fed dinner to residents, assisted them in the bathroom and into bed, checked their insulin levels, and performed a slew of other tasks such as documentation and passing out medications. They tried to control residents' dementia symptoms, but on this night the dementia unit transformed from relative quiet to barely controlled chaos. Bud was one of the most agitated residents. He persistently tried to wheel into residents' rooms and slam the doors closed; he spit into his hands; he ate mayonnaise directly from the packets; and he tried to open the food cart, which was filled with dirty trays. Stephanie tried a number of ways to stop Bud, and one point she walked past me and whispered, "He knows what he is doing," because he smirked at her repeatedly. Later that night, he smacked Jamie, a petite nursing assistant in her early twenties, in the face and laughed. It was not the smack that bothered her as much as the laughing, because the laughter was evidence, in her mind, that he hit her intentionally. A few days later I interviewed Stephanie and asked her about that night. She explained, "When I know somebody's doing something on purpose, that's when they'll get under my skin, you know, and the gentleman the other night, he knows what he's doing. I mean, yes, they do have dementia, not everything they do they realize but—especially when the gentleman, you know, he does it and he smirks and he laughs about it. And, you know, you'll say please not to do—you know, please don't do that and then, you know, he'll look right at you, smirk, and do it again. That frustrates me." After Bud hit Jamie, Joanne organized the training from the Alzheimer's Association. The three-hour training was coming to an end when Jamie spoke up and asked, almost rhetorically, why she had been hit by Bud because she had not done anything wrong and could not comprehend why he would do that to her. This began a lengthy discussion that reframed the event to be consistent with the denial, or at least the justification, of agency.

The trainer asked Jamie to recall the brain images she displayed earlier and noted that Bud did not understand what he had done. Jamie disagreed because after Bud smacked her he began laughing, which in her mind suggested he knew exactly what he had done. She told the group he hit her so hard her ears rang for days. As various members of the staff spoke about Bud's disruptive behavior, the trainer refocused the discussion by calling on me. Out of about twenty people in the conference room, I was the only man, and she ostensibly wanted to get inside the mind of a man. She turned to me and asked how I would have reacted if I was Bud, and I hesitantly said, "I don't know because I don't have dementia." Nervous that I was going to "contaminate the data," I did not want to say anything at all. But she pressed and told me to answer as if I did not have dementia. She asked, "How would you feel if someone was coming in your room, and it was the middle of the night, pitch black, and here you are in a strange place with an alarm going off?" I replied, "Embarrassed, scared," and the instructor cut me off and loudly reiterated "Scared!" and in a very animated tone said Bud hit Jamie not because Bud is a bad person but because he was scared and "needed to be in control." A stranger, Jamie, had entered his room and fear took over; thus his violent reaction was like an instinct and not his fault. She reiterated that staff members needed to be mindful about how they approached residents, and she asked the staff how they could approach Bud differently to lead him to comply with care. Her point was clear: Bud may have intentionally struck Jamie, but given the entirety of the situation, it was not his fault; Jamie should have approached Bud differently.

The denial of responsibility is largely independent of whether residents "truly" intended to strike the staff; rather, it is much more dependent upon staff emotional needs. In the staff members' stories, as in accounts more generally, human agency is denied with justifications and excuses, and those denials deflect blame.[19] But the staff members' accounts of residents' behavior are deployed not to deflect blame, but to maintain sympathy for others. In doing so, residents remain worthy of care. The accounts are a staff rhetorical strategy to manage themselves and their emotions while performing intimate labor.

Agency is not only a theoretical construct, but also a moral—and pragmatic—concept, used as a resource and deployed in the process of making meaning. Over and over I listened to shocking stories of physical, verbal, and even sexual assaults. The staff endured these outbursts without anger or regret so long as they believed such events to be unintentional and not the willful action of a mean, angry individual who was unworthy of care. Making attributions about the agency of residents was an essential element in that process. The floor staff and the managers resisted seeing negative emotional states, such as aggression, as part of being who someone "truly" was. Scholars have noted how people define certain emotional states as negative and then work to transform them.[20] For the staff to find their work satisfying and meaningful, they had to maintain a sense of doing care work that was wanted and appreciated on individuals who were worthy of their care. If staff thought residents were intentionally slapping, kicking, and scratching, such thoughts would undermine their sense of doing meaningful, dignified work that helped people who could not help themselves. The denial of human agency was a rhetorical tool to "redeem" the resident. When individuals were suffering from dementia symptoms and at the end of their lives, the staff did not want to think of them as bad people. Therefore, they used a mechanism of redemption that denied agency and saved them from having to tell stories that did not fit the norm.[21] In the process, staff redeemed themselves.

Nursing home care workers used a rhetoric of agency as a resource to make sense of, and manage tensions in, their work. Their attributions of intent constructed a locally shared moral order in which sympathetic staff attended compassionately to the needs of deserving, dignified residents under the caring roof of a nursing home. The staff invoked agency around death and denied the agency of unruly residents. These findings run counter to those of Gubrium, who argued that dying residents "waited to die" and aggressive residents were routinely chemically and physically restrained because their actions were thought to be intentional.[22] What accounts for these changes in the attribution of agency?

Ascriptions made by nursing home care workers at Rolling Hills and Golden Bay were supported by recent trends in professional philosophies around dying and dementia. The hospice movement recognizes active dying as a set of physiological changes when death is near and emphasizes the role of "letting go" among patients when they die.[23] Hospice developed into a modern coherent philosophy during the 1960s, and its central idea that dying can be a dignified, comfortable, and even joyous end to life has been incorporated into nursing home care.[24] In recent decades, the number of hospices has declined but the number of people in hospice care at nursing homes has steadily increased, and hospice has been integrated into the structure of nursing home care.

Similarly, current scientific thought about the etiology of dementia centers on impaired brain functioning.[25] Patients are viewed as unable to control or even understand their behavior due to circumstances out of their control, and this was emphasized in staff interactions and shown vividly during the Alzheimer's Association training at Rolling Hills. The staff were encouraged to visualize degenerated brain tissue to frame aggressive behavior sympathetically, much like the flight attendants in Hochschild's study who were instructed to imagine belligerent passengers as fearful and childlike.[26] These interpretive frames contribute to organizational stability. The organizational cultivation of sympathy for violent residents managed the floor staff because it mitigated the potential for staff to retaliate against residents. If staff viewed aggressive outbursts as intentional, retaliation could be plausibly constructed as self-defense. Given the terrible history of institutional abuses against vulnerable populations, allegations of mistreatment represent an enormous risk that is reduced by attributing bad behavior as unintentional. Moreover, the social organization of death as something the staff has little control over reduces the considerable potential for stress and emotional burnout.[27] If resident deaths were constructed as something the skilled care could prevent, then dying could be conceived as the result of poor care. Last, if staff felt residents intentionally struck them, they might make demands on their employers for protection, and insist the facility not accept residents with a history of violent behavior.

The reimbursement and regulatory structure of nursing home care also plays a role in the way staff make these attributions. The Nursing Home Reform Act of 1987 inadvertently created a financial incentive for management to screen for, and accept, individuals with a history of violence. Medicare and Medicaid reimburse more when residents have documented verbal, physical, or sexual outbursts. Prior to the 1987 reforms, the federal payment structure for long-term care did not take such behaviors into account when reimbursement rates were calculated. At Rolling Hills and Golden Bay, floor staff said that managers admitted poorly behaved residents because it increased reimbursements, without regard to the impact such residents had on the nursing assistants. The cultivation of sympathy toward aggressive residents helped to insulate the management from these allegations, while boosting revenue and forestalling demands from staff for protection.

Furthermore, the Nursing Home Reform Act put substantial restrictions on the use of chemical or physical restraints to subdue unruly residents. Prior to the legislation, restraint use was prevalent and widely varied across facilities.[28] Staff at both nursing homes who recalled the era before the act said restraints were used routinely as a form of care. The legislation strongly discouraged restraint use and prohibited nursing homes from using them unless a physician ordered them, and it established residents' right to be free of restraints for the purposes of discipline or convenience. According to a report by the Kaiser Family Foundation twenty years after the Nursing Home Reform Act, restraint use dropped from about 40 percent prior to 1987 to less than 6 percent in 2007.[29] The dramatic changes in the way agency has been attributed and denied to residents are consistent with changes in the social organization of nursing home care put forth in the Nursing Home Reform Act, particularly in collaboration with recent professional philosophies, trainings, and staff interactions at Rolling Hills and Golden Bay. In this respect, attributions of intent shape, and are shaped by, a historically situated, locally shared, moral order.

More generally, agency is a cultural object whose use is subject to empirical inquiry. People construct meaning from experience though a social process of attribution. This extends our understanding of agency out of the abstract realm of theoretical construct and into the empirical realm of social interaction. My argument extends beyond the case of nursing care workers presented here, not least to sociology itself. Attributions of agency are shaped and constrained by available interpretive frames. Different frames have different, overlapping logics; thus, the general processes to attribute agency may be universal, but they manifest uniquely based upon particular social conditions. Much like nursing assistants, sociologists deploy agency as a rhetorical resource. Sociologists often use attributions of agency to make arguments that rest on no more or less evidence than nursing home staff who insisted that Mabel controlled her death and that Bud did not control his outbursts. Sociological debates around inequality, deviance, and social movements, among many others, are organized around understandings of agency as if it were something that people possess. My analysis here suggests that we could as profitably look at the ways sociologists deploy the concept of agency—to what ends and under what conditions—as we look at the way others deploy the concept. We would, then, be well served to think about agency itself sociologically—as a set of understandings ascribed to a set of behaviors, used to create and grasp moral meanings in social life and to come to terms, in a variety of ways, with those meanings.

8

Connecting Quality of Life and Quality of Work

As workplaces, nursing homes offer few rewards. The pay and prestige are low, the prospects of career advancement are slim, and the decline and death of the customers are routinized into the fabric of care. Nursing home care workers, even the managers, have very little autonomy over their work routines and often find themselves doing care work tasks in ways that satisfy the demands of their organizations instead of meeting the needs of their residents. The payment and regulatory structures that shape the character of the nursing home industry perpetuate the difficulties that workers face on the job. Faced with workplace conditions that constrain care workers, the staff who do not leave for better jobs often turn to the symbolic to make work feel meaningful. They use emotional labor to build attachments to residents that seem outside of the structure of care, and in doing so, those emotions control residents' behaviors in ways that make their work bearable. They make selective attributions of agency to position residents as worthy of care.

There were important differences between the two nursing homes, including their approaches to admissions, staffing practices, and the outcomes of their health and safety inspections. These differences are consistent with the literature showing that nonprofit nursing homes provide better care than for-profit nursing homes on a wide range of measures.[1] Similarly, popular resources like *Consumer Reports* recommend that nursing home customers are more likely to get better nursing home care at an independently owned nonprofit as opposed to a for-profit chain. I expected to find differences between the two nursing homes along the lines shown in prior research. What I did not expect to find was that their differences would be overshadowed by their similarities.

The two nursing homes were so similar because they operated within a structural context that turns nursing home residents into the embodiment of reimbursable activities, incentivizes nursing homes to make residents more dependent on staff, and normalizes understaffing and work overload. Nonprofits are particularly constrained because they operate within a reimbursement system that undermines mission-oriented business practices. We should want all nursing homes to admit residents without regard to their payer source, but we saw how this practice took Rolling Hills to the brink of financial ruin. Of the $151 billion spent on nursing home care in 2012, Medicaid paid $46 billion, residents and families paid $43 billion directly out of pocket, Medicare paid $34 billion, private insurance paid $12 billion, and charitable donations paid for $11 billion (the remaining $5 billion come from a range of programs such as workers' compensation and the Department of Veterans Affairs).[2] Rolling Hills' finances showed a similar spread of funding; less than 5 percent of their revenue came from charitable donations. Considering that so little nursing home revenue comes from charitable donations, within a payment structure that works to the advantage of for-profits, it is no wonder that nonprofits like Rolling Hills have to adopt some of the policies and practices of their for-profit counterparts. A recent review article concluded similarly, "Even those whose research has consistently found for-profit versus nonprofit cost and quality differences point out that nonprofits are forced to adopt for-profit strategies in competitive markets to compete."[3] Rolling Hills and Golden Bay are, in this sense, case studies in the social-structural processes that generate organizational similarity, or institutional isomorphism.

The concern that nonprofits would be eviscerated by the rise in for-profit health services organizations did not materialize, but that does not tell us much about the relative health or value of the nonprofit sector.[4] The institutional structure of care rewards behaviors consistent with for-profit care and imposes limits on nonprofit altruistic activities. Furthermore, given the federal reporting devices used to measure nursing home quality, it is very difficult to ascertain the unique benefits that nonprofit facilities bring to communities because they do not measure community engagement or charitable care. This is made harder by an institutional structure that weakens the latitude of nonprofits to operate in the public interest. Recall the drop-in center that Rolling Hills subsidized. Funding the center was an important community activity, but Rolling Hills was not recognized by the Centers for Medicare and Medicaid Services (CMS) for providing this service. The CMS does not do enough to encourage and reward these business practices, and in fact their reimbursement and regulatory policies constrain such activities. These are the types of activities that should be rewarded, not discouraged. Given the intense competition nonprofits face from their for-profit competitors, within a reimbursement structure that rewards volume over value, nonprofit nursing homes like Rolling Hills face substantial difficulty fully adopting a mission orientation. Without a profit margin, it's difficult to engage in substantial altruistic activities.[5]

The Minimum Data Set (MDS) form brings this structure into practice. It is the federal reporting device used to assess nursing home residents and monitor their care. The MDS was implemented as part of the 1987 Nursing Home Reform Act to better monitor the care of nursing home residents. The MDS orients nursing home care toward the quantification of care practices and procedures that undermine a holistic approach to quality of life for residents. Of the twenty-four "quality indicators" on the MDS form, only two are related to quality of life.[6] Furthermore, staff assessments of nursing homes are not correlated strongly with residents' self-assessments.[7] The complex and tedious documentation required for regulatory and reimbursement systems, particularly since the Nursing Home Reform Act, has produced a system of "paper compliance." Recent scholarship has noted the preponderance of paper compliance, something that comes very close to what I saw at Golden Bay and Rolling Hills: "Workers respond to pressure to provide quality care by underreporting problems and documenting service levels that are not met and care plans that are not honored because they lack effective feasible interventions and because surveyors rely so heavily on MDS and medical chart reviews."[8] I would add that reimbursements go up with paper compliance. As we have seen, nursing homes are very concerned that all care performed is documented, while documenting care that was not completed is less of a problem for the managers. If care performed is not documented, the facility has missed the reimbursement money. If care is documented but not performed, the facility has gained reimbursement money for work that was not done. The system runs directly opposite to how it should work.

Policies that measure care through aggregate health outcomes collected by the MDS examine quality of life along the margins and create financial opportunities for organizations to routinize care with as few staff members as possible, placing operational efficiency at the center of residents' and workers' experiences. This leads to mechanical, bureaucratized, and impersonal care at a time when residents need personal attention—medically and socially—to a perhaps greater extent than at any other time in their lives. The unique needs of nursing home residents can become a problem or a nuisance to be managed because they hinder operational efficiency. This is not the fault of individual nursing homes or care workers, as the financial problems at Rolling Hills made clear that the problem is systemic. Nursing homes have few viable options other than to operate like Golden Bay, with a business model effectively no different from one used, as Ruby put it, to purchase clothes from a department store.

In this early stage of what will be enormous growth in the elderly population who need long-term care, it is time to rethink the regulatory, financial, legal, and organizational frameworks that structure nursing home care, because they encourage nursing homes to make residents as dependent as possible on as few staff members as possible. These frameworks undermine the relations between care workers and care recipients. Facilities invest operational resources in the departments that are essential to physical health like nursing and rehabilitation, while departments responsible for residents' social lives and emotional health are underfunded by design.

Taken together, the financial and regulatory structures create a model of care in nursing homes that rewards a high volume of instrumental acts of nursing care properly documented, while devaluing the emotional and social components of care work. Nursing homes are reimbursed more when residents are more dependent on staff with their daily care routines. This is no small matter. We have a system of health care financing and regulation that encourages nursing homes to treat residents as if they are entirely dependent. Nursing homes should promote functional independence and wellness and should be rewarded for that; instead, the reality is the other way around. This affects the residents, of course, but it also affects the staff. Recall, for example, how Frankie's coworkers complained that he worked too slowly because he allowed residents to care for themselves as much as possible. Although Frankie was correct that part of rehabilitation is to encourage residents to do as much for themselves as possible, in practice his coworkers were doing what their managers wanted and what the reimbursement system rewarded: to provide more care faster and with fewer resources. There are many residents in nursing homes who, if given enough time, could perform some daily aspects of care independently. But chronic understaffing and work overload force nursing assistants to rush, especially on the day shift, and they do not have the time to be patient with residents, let alone provide the emotional care they would benefit from at the end of life.[9] That works to the financial advantage of the facility and to the disadvantage to the workers and the residents. Nursing homes should be rewarded when they restore or sustain residents' abilities to care for themselves.

One of the ways the reimbursement structure could be changed to improve nursing home quality would be to restructure Medicare and Medicaid to reimburse facilities for value instead of volume. The Patient Protection and Affordable Care Act makes changes along these lines for hospital reimbursements but not for nursing homes. Rather than reimburse on the basis of the amount of therapy and daily assistance provided to residents, Medicaid and Medicare could pay more for better outcomes such as lower rates of pressure ulcers and better staff-resident ratios. Currently reimbursements overlook the activities, social services, and dietary services departments that are essential to enhancing residents' quality of life. They could offer reimbursements to nursing homes that have strong volunteer networks, or involve residents in meal planning, or have activities on every unit every day. In other words, the incentive system should be geared toward improving the quality of life for residents instead of paying on the basis of quantity of reimbursable procedures and treatment. This is precisely what the Medicare Payment Advisory Commission called for in a recent report to Congress.[10] An even bolder solution is to fully federalize the Medicaid program and combine the payment systems so that there is no reason for nursing homes to seek out Medicare residents and treat Medicaid residents as second-class customers. There is no good reason why nursing homes should be paid less for treating poor elderly on Medicaid. This change would likely raise Medicaid payments and lower Medicare payments. Considering that the nursing home industry is bifurcated between resource-poor nursing homes that have very few Medicare payers and lucrative facilities that make a lot of money from Medicare, equalizing Medicare and Medicaid payments would go far toward raising the overall standard of nursing home care.[11]

The Culture Change Movement

There are other important changes that could be made to nursing home care that would enhance resident quality of life while also improving the lives of staff who work in nursing homes.[12] It is regrettable that scholars and policy makers have only recently noted the deep and abiding connections.[13] There are powerful institutional pressures on nursing homes to treat residents as if they exist according to the extent that they embody reimbursable activities. As this dynamic has intensified, many elder care practitioners have coalesced into something of a "movement" to improve the culture of nursing homes. The "culture change movement" encompasses a variety of different ideas championed by a number of different organizations, advocates, and policy makers that promote "person-centered" or "person-directed" care for the elderly. In the culture change model, elders ideally have much of the same privacy and choices they would have living in their own home. The Pioneer Network, an advocacy organization of nursing home care practitioners that began the movement, describes the core values of culture change as "choice, dignity, respect, self-determination and purposeful living."[14] Although the culture change movement involves a number of organizations and can take a variety of particular forms, they coalesce in the following six domains: (1) resident-directed care and activities; (2) a living environment that is more like a home than a hospital; (3) close relationships between residents and their family, staff, and community members; (4) empowered staff members; (5) decentralized decision making; and (6) continuous quality improvement based on measured and comprehensive outcomes.[15] The overarching goal is the transformation of the nursing home from operating based on an institutional-bureaucratic logic, what I have referred to as a logic of cost, to a logic of care that puts the individuals living in nursing homes at the center of all practices and priorities—to make a home out of an institution.

Some organizations aligned with the culture change movement advocate for the creation of smaller, home-like buildings that have common living spaces and private bedrooms in which residents live on their own schedules. These facilities, based on what is known as the green house model, are staffed by a small number of nursing assistants who have received additional training and have greater autonomy and are known as "Shahbazim."[16] They manage the household and are supported by nurses and rehabilitation therapists. Another model of culture change is known as the Eden alternative; this model endorses gardens, companion animals, frequent visits from children, and even innovations as straightforward as replacing white towels and linens with brightly colored ones to give a more lively appearance to existing facilities. Still a third model of culture change, the Wellspring model, is followed by a network of nonprofit nursing homes based in Wisconsin that work together to improve resident care through greater empowerment of nursing assistants and other staff members who perform direct care. Staff members are trained in nationally recognized best care practices and can consult with interdisciplinary "care-resource teams" when needed. The nursing homes in the network share information to improve care, with the goal a keeping residents at the center of their concerns.

The rapid growth in various forms of culture change initiatives and the efforts under way to implement those changes are encouraging signs that the nursing home industry understands that it can do more to improve the lives of the elderly. But these efforts are constrained by the structural context of nursing home care.[17] Consider a recent Commonwealth Fund study that found that cost, scope, and regulatory structure were significant barriers to implementing culture change.[18] Similarly, a report by the National Commission for Quality Long Term Care found that culture change was "swimming against a tide of regulation, limited resources, and established practices."[19] Recently the CMS has provided modest institutional support for culture change implementation, but this agency could do more to modify the regulatory and reimbursement policies to be centered around residents instead of operational efficiencies.[20] The structural context of nursing home care prevents deep, systemic changes to the industry. There will be no broad-based cultural change absent major structural change.

The perceived barriers to culture change implementation vary depending on familiarity with its principles.[21] Those most familiar with culture change said resistance by senior management was the number one barrier and those least familiar cited cost as preventing culture change implementation. Furthermore, nursing home care workers are almost three times as likely as other long-term care staff such as home care aids to cite the regulatory system as the number one barrier to implementation. The study concluded, "To promote adoption, research and broad-based educational efforts are needed to influence views and perceptions. Fundamental changes in the regulatory process together with targeted regulatory changes and payment incentives may also be needed."[22] Many nursing home care workers are eager to improve the conditions of care but are constrained by the regulatory and reimbursement structures, which are organized around an institutional-bureaucratic logic that undermines attention to residents' quality of daily life.

The culture change movement is intended to improve not only the quality of residents' lives, but also the quality of staff members' work lives. Empowering nursing assistants, a core element in the culture change movement, is a key component to improving care. A recent study, for example, found that when nursing assistants were included in decision-making processes, nursing home residents had a lower incidence of pressure ulcers and were more involved in social activities.[23] In addition, management practices that are more inclusive and less authoritative are related to better resident outcomes in a number of areas including a lower use of physical restraints and a lower incidence of aggressive behaviors among residents.[24] Another recent study found that nursing home residents were more satisfied with their quality of life on units where a higher proportion of nursing assistants were committed to their work.[25]

Rolling Hills and Golden Bay had ambivalent positions toward implementing the values that make up the culture change movement. Virtually all the managers at both facilities had heard of it and supported the goal of person-centered care. But they were so entrenched in their daily routines that making changes that were more than cosmetic, particularly if they cost money, did not seem worth the effort. For example, Liz returned from a meeting that introduced culture change principles to activities directors and was excited by what she learned. The meeting changed the way she saw her role in the facility. Before she had concentrated on getting new residents accustomed to life in institutional care. After attending the meeting, she explained, "I feel like I've been institutionalizing people." Now she wanted to do more to enable residents to be as independent as possible. She planned to get a small kitchenette installed in a corner of the main dining room where residents could, say, make themselves a cup of tea or coffee at their own leisure. She knew that her department's budget of just a few hundred dollars a month could not absorb the costs, and she did not bother to ask Andy for extra money. She did get information about a funding grant she could apply for, but she did not have the time or the knowledge and skills to write a grant proposal herself. Also, Andy was concerned that installing a kitchenette would require staff to be off the unit and watching any resident who used it, because if anyone were injured it would surely lead to problems with the state. To my knowledge she never submitted the grant application. Rolling Hills did, however, change her title to the more culture change appropriate "life enhancement leader." Golden Bay approached culture change the same way. Although they maintained the steep top-town hierarchy that kept nursing assistants from meaningful participation in decision making at any level in the organization, they made superficial changes that gave a nod to the culture change movement. For instance, they renamed the different units after local towns so that instead of saying that a resident was going to "unit two" it sounded as if they were headed to a nearby town.

These cosmetic adjustments as a form of culture change are quite common, according to a recent study by the Commonwealth Fund.[26] The researchers found that almost 70 percent of nursing homes surveyed reported that they had implemented culture change not at all or only in a few respects. They also found wide variation in the extent that nursing homes were implementing culture change principles that foster resident-centered care, such as allowing residents to determine their own daily schedule or involving residents in organizational decision making. Only about 15 percent of nursing homes reported that their nursing assistants worked in self-managed teams or were cross-trained for multiple functional roles in the workplace. However, the study also found that as nursing homes adopted culture change principles, staff retention, resident occupancy rates, market competitiveness, and operational costs improved. The study does not say anything about why progress in transforming nursing homes from institutions to homes has been slow, but my research certainly offers a powerful answer. Nursing homes will do more to implement culture change principles when the reimbursement and regulatory systems make it worth the investment of time, energy, and money. Nursing homes are constrained in what they can do given the structural context around them. Without structural changes, efforts at cultural change are likely to fall flat.

Nursing assistants who are empowered with knowledge and greater autonomy—core principles of the culture change movement—provide better care for residents and have better working conditions that improve upon the problems that have traditionally plagued nursing homes. A recent study compared nursing assistants who worked together in a team-based care work approach and those who did not and concluded that "the empowered work teams had positive impacts on CNA performance by allowing the CNAs to become more aware of resident health conditions, by providing them with more information on the special care needs of residents, by giving them the opportunity to question the poor performance of negligent team members, by giving them the time needed to clear up misinformation and communication, and because the team members were more willing to carry out decisions that they participated in making."[27]

The point here is that the quality of care is deeply connected to the quality of work. Nursing assistants are organizationally positioned to have the most knowledge about residents' preferences. They know what residents want when they wake up in the morning and before they go to bed, what they like to wear, and what kinds of food they like to eat. Nursing assistants are often the first to notice changes in residents' behavior that could indicate changes in health or behavioral status. They are in the best position to make decisions regarding residents' daily care routines, and when they are empowered to do so, care becomes less routine and more personal and thrives on close relationships between residents and staff.[28] Yet understaffing and organizational inertia limit the participation of nursing assistants in resident care planning.

One might think that team-based care would be a core component of the culture change movement. Team-based care work, however, is the least often implemented component among nursing homes that are implementing culture change principles, suggesting that nursing homes have difficulty moving away from a hierarchical job structure despite the evidence that doing so improves staff satisfaction and resident quality of life.[29] A recent analysis suggests that teamwork is closely associated with organizational culture.[30] Nursing homes with high teamwork were more likely to attribute positive motivations to their colleagues such as a love of the elderly or a desire to work hard. These facilities also had managers who modeled information exchange, worked on the units with staff, and regularly provided feedback to staff. Nursing homes with low teamwork tended to attribute negative motivations to their colleagues, suggesting that they worked with the elderly only for the flexible schedule or the money and had managers who did not model teamwork and other forms of resident-centered care.

Cultivating Emotions

In addition to changes to the culture of nursing homes, there need to be changes to the structure of workplace practices if nursing homes will be better suited to the needs and desires of the elderly. One way to do this would be to cultivate opportunities for emotional authenticity between staff and residents.[31] My research has shown that even despite structural obstacles that undermine emotions, workers found opportunities to connect with residents and used emotional labor as a skill to generate dignity and meaning. An organizational and regulatory framework that supports a culture of emotional authenticity in nursing home care would improve both the quality of work and the quality of life in nursing homes. After all, the average length of stay in a nursing home is nearly two and a half years. Nursing home residents can enjoy the benefits of connecting with others even if those others are being paid to care. Nursing assistants feel attached to residents, and those attachments are some of the most important reasons they stay in the field.

If nursing homes were to cultivate opportunities for authentic emotional attachments between staff and residents, perhaps it would lower staff turnover, which is very high.[32] Emotional attachments are important to workers. A recent nationally representative survey of nursing assistants conducted by the Centers for Disease Control and Prevention found that 50 percent of respondents said that the main reason they continue to work in nursing homes is "caring for others," while only 4 percent said "good pay," 4 percent said "benefits," and 2 percent said "career opportunities." This evidence reinforces the patterns I observed, as nursing assistants claimed over and over that they stayed on the job because they "loved" their residents more than they disliked the low pay and low autonomy. There are likely selection effects; workers who feel compelled by caring for the elderly make careers as nursing assistants, while those who do not eventually cycle out and enter other occupations. Nevertheless, nursing assistants construct emotionally authentic connections to residents. Ann Swidler conceives of culture as a "toolkit" from which individuals use an array of culture repertoires—ways of speaking—as "tools" that we use to construct meaning and manage interactions.[33] Nursing home care workers drew from emotional repertoires as a resource to craft a sense of dignity at work. Workers are not passive victims of social structure; rather, they actively push back against the challenges they confront as they endeavor to create meaning in their everyday activities. For nursing home care workers, emotions are, to paraphrase Swidler, a power tool.

The framework of emotions I have developed here, in which workers use emotions as a rhetorical resource to construct dignity, contrasts to some degree with Hochschild's theory of emotional labor.[34] Emotional labor is most applicable to workers who have a high volume of brief interactions with customers regarding largely impersonal concerns. In the long-term interactions between floor staff and residents, managers were less able to control interactions and workers were more able to shape how they unfolded. Imagine a plane ride that lasted as long as the average length of stay in a nursing home, two and a half years. How long would it take for the standard scripts between flight attendants and passengers to break down? The production of emotional labor is less relevant for the increasing number of workers who have face-to-face interactions with individuals over long periods of time. Nursing home care workers at Rolling Hills and Golden Bay moved within the boundaries that structure care work to carve out spaces of emotional authenticity. While the emotional labor perspective highlights the role of emotions in the reproduction of organizational goals, I found that emotions acted as a symbolic resource turned to the purposes of personal goals. Emotional labor encourages discipline and compliance to organizations. The emotional labor that I witnessed among nursing home care workers in some ways undermined organizational goals because it ran counter to the operational efficiencies that standardize care. In a few cases, closeness to residents led staff members to provide care that went against the directives of managers, actively resisting their efforts based on the extent they cared about residents. On the other hand, they also bonded workers to particular residents in ways that could result in an "emotional hostage effect," in which paid care workers developed close personal relationships with residents that kept them working in bad jobs.[35] Ultimately, emotional attachments that *felt authentic* were at the center of how staff crafted dignity at work.

Workers claim a dignified identity built upon caring for and about others.[36] Amid structural and institutional constraints that weaken workers' autonomy and power in the workplace, they struggle to achieve a sense of purpose. The context of low wages, low prestige, and low autonomy pushes workers toward alternative hierarchies of meaning that give their work value. Sociologist Michele Lamont argued that among the working class, "moral standards function as an alternative to economic definitions of success and offer them a way to maintain dignity and to make sense of their lives in a land where the American dream is ever more out of reach."[37] In order to draw dignity from work amid increasing inequality, those toward the bottom of the class system who are unlikely to achieve material wealth turn to moral and symbolic means to measure their self-worth. Workers construct symbolic hierarchies to position themselves above others, below whom they reside on more traditional grounds of wealth, status, and authority.[38] This is how workers in devalued occupations, particularly those who have extended interactions with customers, craft dignity at work. Dignity is a relational concept, constructed with a kind of self-evaluation in reference to a generalized other.[39] It is likely that workers in health care and education whose work entails extended interactions with others, often in situations that create opportunities for authentic emotional attachments, experience a sense of meaning and dignity through these interactions. For these and a growing number of service occupations such as child care workers, teachers, and therapists, using emotions as a resource is a critical part of the job. It is time to recognize, cultivate, and encourage those emotions.

Where Do We Go from Here?

Every day for the next twenty years, more than ten thousand people in the United States will turn sixty-five, and we have only begun to prepare for the long-term care challenges these individuals will present. Right now more than 5 million people over the age of sixty-five use long-term care services, and about 1.8 million of them live in nursing homes. These numbers will increase sharply over the next thirty years. The Department of Health and Human Services (DHHS) projects that, if residency rates remain stable, the number of people living in nursing homes will double by 2030 and triple for people over the age of eighty-five. Even if the residency rates decline substantially (meaning more people get round-the-clock care at home), the DHHS projects that the number of people in nursing homes will rise by at least 57 percent, about nine hundred thousand more people. Unpaid family caregivers assist the vast majority of individuals who currently need long-term care. For a variety of reasons, unpaid care work in the home will not be able to meet the growing need for long-term care. Of the people who get long-term care whose services are paid for, Medicaid is the largest provider. This is important because Medicaid covers individuals only after they have exhausted their financial resources and have very minimal incomes. The long-term care industry takes the life savings of far too many people, draining their financial resources until there is virtually nothing left.

Medicaid was designed to pay for the care of the poor and the disabled, but it does more than that. It is a program that many middle-class and relatively affluent families rely on for long-term care in nursing homes. Many middle-class families do not know that Medicaid will likely pay the nursing home bills of their parents and grandparents. Medicaid protects middle-class families as the bedrock program that pays for nursing home care, even though it was not intended to be that program. We imagine that Medicaid covers only poor people, but in fact it is a key part of the social safety net for middle-class families whose needs for nursing home care outlast their financial resources to pay for that care.

The Patient Protection and Affordable Care Act left the emerging challenge of long-term care in America largely unaddressed, except for one provision known as the Community Living Assistance Services and Supports Act (CLASS). CLASS was intended to supplement private long-term care insurance by providing a cash benefit of about seventy-five dollars per day (twenty-seven thousand dollars annually) to help pay for long-term care for the disabled and elderly. Working adults would be eligible to participate in this voluntary insurance program. Those individuals would enroll through their employer and pay a monthly premium determined based on age, without regard to health status. After a five-year vesting period, people who developed a functional disability would receive the daily cash benefit. The idea was to help people live at home with a disability or dementia longer than they do now, which would not only cost less than nursing home care but also be more comfortable for most beneficiaries. The benefit could have been used to pay for a wide range of services, including payments to family members to provide care, the installation of wheelchair ramps at home, and nursing home care.

CLASS was an earnest attempt to deal with the impending long-term care crisis the country will face as the population continues to age. Unfortunately, it was repealed during the "fiscal cliff" negotiations in January 2013. The Affordable Care Act required CLASS to be fully self-financed, with premiums and benefits matched to keep the program financially sound for seventy-five years. Given the absence of an individual mandate for the program, enrollments in CLASS were voluntary, making it very difficult to predict how many people would sign up and how much the premiums would need to be given the level of benefits to be paid out to enrollees. Although getting CLASS passed as part of the Affordable Care Act was one of Ted Kennedy's final accomplishments, many politicians opposed it and the Obama administration put it on the chopping block during budget negotiations with the Republican-led House of Representatives.

The demise of CLASS highlights the substantial financial challenges of paying for long-term care, but there are challenges that extend beyond the financial. The question is how we as a country are going to care for the people who will need it. A large number of those people will live at home for longer than used to be the case, but there is a limit to the amount of care that can be provided at home. We have to think more broadly about what we want for our parents, our grandparents, our spouses, and ourselves when long-term care becomes necessary. Changing the culture of nursing homes is a fine starting point, but little change is possible given the current reimbursement and regulatory structure. It is that structure that needs dramatic change if we wish to provide better, more humane care during life's twilight.

From the Poorhouse to the Skilled Nursing Facility

The nursing home care system is fragmented in ways that reflect the American health care system more generally. Medicaid, which was intended originally to provide health insurance for the poor and disabled, has become the primary payment model of nursing home care for the elderly. To understand precisely the confluence of events that produced such a system, this appendix examines the historical trajectory of the nursing home industry and its connections to the politics and policy of health care in the United States.

As the Industrial Revolution progressed throughout the nineteenth century, children increasingly left the family home and migrated to emerging urban centers in order to find work. This was a profound change in family structure that left older adults without the assistance they needed, and once had, to live at home into old age. Public welfare policies at the time were modeled on the English Poor Laws that established a very limited government role to provide assistance for dependent individuals who could not care for themselves.[1] The scope and implementation of assistance for the elderly and indigent were left to local counties and municipalities, not federal authorities, and county "poorhouses" and "poor farms" emerged across a young America to house the poor elderly. Poorhouses provided meager housing and support to elderly individuals who could not work enough to afford rent or otherwise support themselves. Poor farms were often working farms whose elderly residents were expected to work in the fields to the extent that their health allowed. Due to public concern that the prospect of free shelter and food would attract individuals pretending to be poor, poorhouses and poor farms were intentionally made unappealing.[2] The elderly lived in fear of the poorhouse, and for good reason. Conditions were deplorable, poorhouse "inmates" were often required to wear uniforms, and by the beginning of the twentieth century poorhouses became the dumping grounds for society's undesirables. Along with the elderly, petty criminals, alcoholics, and the mentally ill filled the poorhouses.

In sharp contrast to the dreadful poorhouse environment, a small nonprofit sector of homes for the elderly emerged. They were typically private homes that were owned and operated by churches, a variety of fraternal organizations, and immigrants who served members of those groups, particularly widows and disabled individuals. These facilities, charitable in nature, became the center of the early nonprofit nursing home industry.[3]

The Great Depression was particularly devastating to the elderly, as millions of retired or nearly retired individuals lost their savings and became completely dependent on their adult children, a historic number of whom were unemployed. The alarming increase in the number of poor elderly and the problematic conditions of poorhouses across the country gave rise to "aging" as a national public issue, as legislators debated how to provide adequate assistance while also discouraging the growth of poorhouses.[4] The federal government became involved in nursing homes for the first time in 1935 with the passage of the Social Security Act, which established a federal and state public assistance program for the elderly poor called Old Age Assistance (OAA). The OAA program provided cash payments to those in need regardless of their work history, but on the condition that benefits be prohibited to anyone who was living in a public institution such as a poorhouse. The intent was to provide the poor elderly with the means to seek better shelter than poorhouses and also to nudge people living in poorhouses to seek housing elsewhere. It worked to great effect, as poorhouse populations declined sharply after 1935 and poorhouses disappeared almost completely by the 1950s.[5]

A new cottage industry of small mom-and-pop proprietary homes for the aged emerged in place of the poorhouses, sparked by the new cash benefit OAA provided. These new shelters were most commonly empty rooms in private homes that could easily generate revenue at a time when millions of people were out of work. Unemployed nurses provided rudimentary care to the sick elderly, giving rise to the term "nursing home." The new proprietary operators emerged alongside the already existing nonprofit charitable facilities, most of which allowed access only to members of their own organizations or immigrant groups. This left proprietary homes with an enormous opportunity; they were the only option for the elderly that accepted OAA benefits and could meet the growing demand for care.[6]

Conditions favorable to the growth of proprietary nursing homes continued in the decades between Roosevelt's New Deal and Johnson's Great Society programs. For one thing, there were a lot of potential customers. Throughout the 1940s, almost 25 percent of the population sixty-five and over received OAA benefits, more than two million people annually. As demand for long-term care services expanded, so did the need for new and larger facilities. Congress passed the Hill-Burton Act in 1940, which provided more than two and a half billion dollars in federal grants and low-interest loans to improve the medical infrastructure over the next twenty-five years.[7] In addition, various amendments to the Social Security Act expanded OAA benefits and allowed for the rapid growth of proprietary nursing homes.[8] In the 1940s, federal legislators voted to increase the cap on OAA payments and the share of the assistance paid by the federal government (the balance would be paid by the states). Later amendments allowed the government to pay nursing home operators directly, providing a much more stable source of income than reliance on poor elderly individuals for timely payments. At this time, the federal government required states to create licensing systems for nursing homes, but set no required minimum standards and made no effort to make certain that states enforced whatever standards were set.

In what has become a familiar pattern, nursing home costs increased faster than the value of government benefits, leading lawmakers in 1956 to eliminate the OAA payment caps to medical providers. Soon thereafter, the government became the largest single payer of nursing home care. The easy money available to build a nursing home and the virtually guaranteed income from OAA benefits attracted entrepreneurs interested in cashing in on old age, setting ripe conditions for massive private investment. These changes created the environment for the emergence of a profit-oriented nursing home industry; predictably, spending on nursing home care increased by 181 percent and the bed supply doubled to over one million in less than a decade.[9]

During this period of rapid growth leading up to the passage of Medicare and Medicaid in 1965, concerns about nursing home safety emerged as a public health issue. Congressional committees and various public health agencies reported that few nursing homes were of adequate quality, that states did not have basic standards or enforcement mechanisms, and that nearly half of nursing home beds across the country failed to meet basic fire and health standards.[10] The Senate Subcommittee on Problems of the Aged and Aging concluded in 1960, "Many states have not fully enforced the existing regulations, failure to do so reflecting the policy of the states to give ample time to the nursing home owners and operators to bring the facilities up to the standards. Many states report that strict enforcement of the regulations would close the majority of homes."[11] It would not be until 1967 that basic federal fire and health regulations were applied to nursing homes.

The passage of the Medicaid and Medicare insurance programs expanded substantially the public funding of nursing home services and gave the federal government authority to set regulatory standards for facilities across the country. Long-term nursing home care was intentionally excluded from Medicare out of fear that its projected costs would ultimately sink the program, financially and politically.[12] Instead, Medicare provided funding for a posthospital recovery period of up to one hundred days (after a qualifying three-night hospital stay) in what would be called an "extended care facility." The short-term coverage provision was included for budgetary purposes, since a day in an extended care facility would cost less than a day in a hospital. The thinking at the time was that getting patients out of hospitals and into postacute recovery facilities would lower overall medical expenditures. Furthermore, lawmakers compromised that the primary focus of Medicare should be insuring curative care in hospitals, not extended custodial care in nursing homes.

At the time, many people believed wrongly (and still do to this day) that Medicare covers long-term care expenses for individuals over the age of sixty-five. It is actually Medicaid that finances most long-term care in the United States, and that is because of a compromise that emerged from Medicare negotiations. Medicaid would provide unlimited coverage of nursing home care, but for only the poorest of the elderly. Those seniors with a net worth above eligibility for the means-tested Medicaid program could access benefits only after they had "spent down" their assets until they had barely anything left. This policy continues to lead to the depletion of the life savings of individuals who require long-term care. Medicaid spending quickly exceeded its cost projections as utilization soared; it became and remains the single greatest purchaser of nursing home services. Nursing homes, which were redefined by Congress as "skilled nursing facilities," would be paid under a fee-for-service model, in which the self-reported costs of care as well as mortgage interest and equipment depreciation were reimbursed by states with matching funds provided by the federal government.[13] The money that flowed from these programs took much of the financial risk out of nursing home care, and the industry exploded. Between 1960 and 1976, the number of nursing homes grew by 140 percent, the number of beds increased by over 300 percent, and industry revenues rose by 2,000 percent, and only a few years later nearly 80 percent of the institutionalized elderly lived in for-profit skilled nursing facilities.[14]

The early 1970s saw a series of high-profile scandals and critical reports about the care provided in nursing homes, forcing the government to react—a repeated pattern in long-term care.[15] Reforms in 1974 were supposed to improve monitoring and increase regulatory enforcement, but they were largely politically symbolic and there was little improvement.[16] Cases of resident mistreatment, neglect, and abuse continued, and public outrage and fear of nursing homes called for a stronger regulatory framework. The nursing home industry never gained the public trust. In 1986 the Institute of Medicine (IOM) issued a report that documented widespread regulatory problems, lackadaisical monitoring, and inconsistent enforcement of the nursing home industry. The report argued for an outcome-based framework, noting that the certification and regulatory process was overly focused on infrastructure capacity and should pay more attention to the quality of services provided.[17] The IOM made a series of recommendations that were largely adopted into law as the Nursing Home Reform Act, part of the Omnibus Budget Reconciliation Act of 1987.

The Nursing Home Reform Act mandated specific requirements for nursing, medical, and mental health training and services, strengthened residents' rights, and introduced a uniform resident assessment instrument for care planning and comprehensive monitoring. Unannounced inspections, an outcome-oriented inspection process, state-appointed ombudsmen as resident advocates, and a wide range of enforcement mechanisms were also key parts of the new law.[18] The *New York Times* editorial pages hailed the legislation and declared, "The act makes clear that residence in a nursing home is not synonymous with a loss of autonomy" and went on to say that the act "guarantees a patient's right to privacy, to voice grievances and to have them promptly addressed" and that "such rights are a comfort to today's nursing home patients and their families."[19] The new regulations have improved care in some ways, especially in the decline in physical restraints use and the increase in nursing home staffing, but serious quality problems persist.[20]

Under pressure to contain rapidly escalating health care costs, in 1997 Congress repealed the law that required Medicaid payments to nursing homes to be "reasonable and adequate," giving states greater freedom to set payment rates, which they lowered immediately.[21] The cycle of scandal and renewed political attention was repeated when, two years later, in the wake of reports of widespread neglect and abuse of California nursing home residents,[22] President Clinton introduced a new round of enforcement mechanisms including harsher fines and unannounced inspections on evenings and weekends. Nevertheless, a follow-up report issued by the IOM on nursing home services continued to recommend tougher standards and enforcement, more penalties, and more data for comprehensive assessment.[23] The report also noted that low Medicaid reimbursement was a potential source of quality deficiencies.

The system continues, and doing more of the same thing—tougher enforcement and harsher penalties—will likely not produce any substantially different results, given the structure upon which the long-term care industry emerged. There was not much coherence or forethought put into the mechanisms by which care for the elderly is delivered and financed, and it is the nursing home residents who pay the price of such a fractured and accidental system.

NOTES

NOTES TO THE INTRODUCTION

1. England, 2005.
2. Sherman, 2007.
3. Bureau of Labor Statistics, 2012a.
4. Evers, Tomic, et al., 2002; Gates, Fitzwater, et al., 2004; Snyder, Chen, et al., 2007.
5. Castle, 2006; Castle and Engberg, 2006.
6. Diamond, 1992; Foner, 1994; Gubrium, 1975; Lopez, 2006a, 2006b.
7. Bureau of Labor Statistics, 2014a, 2014b.
8. Williams, 1992.
9. Bureau of Labor Statistics, 2012b.
10. Federal Interagency Forum on Aging Related Statistics, 2010; He, Sengupta, et al., 2005.
11. Denzin, 1989.
12. Kaffenberger, 2001; Kassirer, 2005; Mahar, 2006.
13. Harrington, Carrillo, et al., 2008; Kaiser Commission on Medicaid and the Uninsured, 2013.
14. Stevenson and Grabowski, 2008.
15. Starr, 1982: 448.
16. Hughes, 1951, 1958.
17. Leidner, 1993.
18. Ashforth and Kreiner, 1999.
19. Schein, 1990; Trice, 1993.
20. Glenn, 2000.
21. Stacey, 2005.
22. Folbre, 2001; Himmelweit, 1999.
23. England, 2005.
24. Diamond, 1992; Foner, 1994; Lopez, 2006b.
25. England, Budig, et al., 2002; Harrington Meyer, 2000.
26. Folbre, 2001; Hochschild, 2013; Stone, 2000.
27. Bowers, Esmond, et al., 2000; Dodson and Zincavage, 2007.
28. Black and Rubinstein, 2005; Moss, Moss, et al., 2003.
29. Duncan and Morgan, 1994; Kemp, Ball, et al., 2009.
30. Dodson and Zincavage, 2007.
31. Bishop, Weinberg, et al., 2008; Hannan, Norman, et al., 2001.

32. Diamond, 1992.
33. Cancian, 2000: 43.
34. Hochschild, 1979.
35. Lee Treweek, 1996; Leidner, 1993; Lopez, 2006b; Paules, 1991; Smith-Lovin, 1998; Tolich, 1993; Wharton, 1993.
36. Hodson, 2001; Hodson and Roscigno, 2004; Lamont, 2000; Sennett, 2009; Sherman, 2007.
37. Gubrium, 1975.

NOTES TO CHAPTER 1

1. See Vladeck (1980) for an example of how these incentives play out at the level of policy.
2. See the appendix for a brief account of the history of institutional care of the poor elderly.
3. Genworth, 2013.
4. Jones, Dwyer, et al., 2009.
5. Swan, Harrington, et al., 2000.
6. Swan, Harrington, et al., 2000.
7. Lipsky, 2010.
8. This reimbursement structure is very similar to how hospitals are now reimbursed. Diagnostic related groupings (DRGs) constitute a system to classify hospital patients into groups that are expected to use a similar amount of resources and expenditures. Payments are based on a fixed amount regardless of the care that is actually required. The DRG system was originally designed to contain Medicare costs, but has expanded and become a way to broadly link categories of patients to the resources they use.
9. The nominal differences in payment are due to Medicaid's policy of adjusting reimbursement rates based on a wide range of variables such as geographical location.
10. Bureau of Labor Statistics, 2008–2009.
11. Collins, Wolf, et al., 2004.
12. Individuals living within the dementia units in nursing homes are most likely to be on Medicaid because they are also most likely to have lived in a nursing home long enough to have spent whatever savings they had paying the facility privately out of pocket until they were poor enough to qualify for Medicaid.
13. On the flow sheet, 2 was a code number to indicate that a moderate level of assistance was provided for a particular activity of daily living.
14. The magnet was used to help stop a seizure. This is an example of when good care lowers overall reimbursement. Everyone knowing how to use a magnet to stop a seizure would make the stopping a seizure more likely, but at the same time it would make seizure control no longer a skilled observation and thus not reimbursable.
15. Walker, 1998.
16. Diamond, 1992; Evans and Porche, 2005.
17. Sykes and Matza, 1957.

18. Evans and Porche, 2005.

19. Mills, 1940.

NOTES TO CHAPTER 2

1. Goffman, 1959: xi.

2. Goffman defined the backstage as "a place, relative to a given performance, where the impression fostered by the performance is knowingly contradicted as a matter of course" (1959: 112). In this space, social actors use a more informal language and may be more apt to relax the impressions they are giving off to others. In the backstage, people can "let their hair down" and "say what they really think," so to speak.

3. Lopez, 2006a.

4. Gubrium, 1975.

5. Levinson, 2008.

6. In the days leading up to Hurricane Katrina, the proprietors of St. Rita's Nursing Home in New Orleans decided not to evacuate the facility. Subsequently, thirty-five residents perished during the storm. The proprietors were charged with and eventually acquitted of the negligent homicide of those who died in their care. The husband and wife owners of the nursing home were the only two people to be tried in criminal court for the incalculable number of mistakes in planning that led to eighteen hundred Katrina-related deaths.

7. The state's reach extends into the backstage as a form of regulatory control over the workplace. This backstage work prepared the facility for frontstage performance, but it is not only that backstage shaped the frontstage. The frontstage, or, to be more precise, the managers' imagination of what would happen in the frontstage, shaped the extent and character of the backstage preparation. This is one sense in which the distinction between backstage and frontstage turns into a hall of mirrors. Similarly, Andy's conversation with the managers was backstage relative to the inspectors but frontstage relative to everyone else in the room.

8. Miller and Mor, 2006.

9. Residents' and Family Councils are two of the reforms implemented by the 1987 Nursing Home Reform Act.

10. Aside from the group interview with inspectors, residents are mostly outside this entire process. Not part of any "team" or "performance," nursing home residents are a curious nonentity in the inspection. Managers viewed the few moments when residents were called upon to act during the inspection as a potential threat to the veracity of the performance, depending on to whom the inspectors were speaking. On rare occasions the savvier residents called the Department of Public Health if they felt their rights had not been honored. Residents usually do not disturb the performance; they normalize to the structure of life in institutional care and likely underreport the extent of actionable grievances.

11. Extended fieldwork presented a multitude of dilemmas. On the one hand, I wanted to gain and reinforce rapport with the staff. On the other hand, I wanted to stay

out of the way and simply observe. This occurred in a moment when there was not much time for reflection or careful consideration of the proper course of action. After spending almost a year observing the facility, I helped Dave, and by extension the nursing home more generally, because I felt like they had helped me so much by allowing me to do research there. If I had not helped them when they needed it, it could have severely harmed my rapport with the staff, and I did not want to take that chance.

12. The 1987 legislation mandated that a nursing home that wanted to physically restrain a resident get a physician's order first. This dramatically reduced the use of restraints on residents (Weiner, Freiman, et al., 2007).

13. Goffman, 1959: 82.

14. Goffman referred to this phenomenon as a "strategic secret." Goffman wrote, "Secrets that are merely strategic tend to be ones which the team eventually discloses, perforce, when action based upon secret preparations is consummated" (1959: 142). In other words, the strategic secrets that give the performance a script, if you will, are an open secret between the staff and the inspectors. These unspoken secrets sustain the interaction and give it a standard progression. All parties involved know the big secret of the "show," and the audience plays along, cocreating the performance.

15. Castle, 2006; Castle and Engberg, 2006.

16. Goffman, 1959: 254.

NOTES TO CHAPTER 3

1. Recent scholarship has looked at the significance of profit status (Amirkhanyan, Kim, et al., 2008; Harrington, Woolhandler, et al., 2001; Hillmer, Wodchis, et al., 2005; O'Neill, Harrington, et al., 2003; Schlesinger and Gray, 2006; Spector, Selden, et al., 1998), size (Verbeek, Zwakhalen, et al., 2010), ownership characteristics (Anderson, Lewis, et al., 1999; Harrington, Woolhandler, et al., 2001; Knox, Blankmeyer, et al., 2001; Martin, O'Meara, et al., 2008; Stevenson and Grabowski, 2008), and whether the facility is located in an urban or rural community (Gessert, Haller, et al., 2006; Penrod, 2001).

2. See http://www.resourcesystems.net/LongTermCare/CareTracker/IncreaseReimbursement.aspx (accessed June 6, 2013).

3. Gubrium, 1986; Pollner and McDonald-Wikler, 1985; Rodriquez, 2009.

4. This was an implicit trust—I trusted that she revealed an accurate picture of how she experienced her work, and she trusted that I would not get her in trouble for anything she revealed.

5. The safety checks were intended to ensure that residents who had difficulty walking independently had a tether between the wheelchair and the resident's shirt. If the resident stood up, an alarm would sound.

6. Gubrium, 1975.

7. Brauer, Coca-Perraillon, et al., 2009.

8. A "tabbed resident" has an alarm clipped onto his or her clothes that is tethered to the wheelchair. If the resident tries to stand up, the alarm sounds. The intent is to prevent falls.

9. Scott-Cawiezell, Jones, et al., 2005.

10. Barry, Brannon, et al., 2005.

11. Barry, Brannon, et al., 2005; Bishop, Squillace, et al., 2009; Bishop, Weinberg, et al., 2008; Pennington, Scott, et al., 2003.

12. Dill, Craft Morgan, et al., 2010; Stone and Harahan, 2010.

13. Horn, Buerhaus, et al., 2005.

14. Scott-Cawiezell, Jones, et al., 2005.

15. Lamont and Molnar, 2002: 168.

16. A recent ethnographic study by Rachel Sherman (2005) analyzed boundary formation in the context of workplace inequality. Luxury hotel workers responded to their subordinate status in the workplace by positioning themselves above their wealthy guests along a range of symbolic, rather than material, hierarchies. Workers crafted a "superior self" by comparing themselves favorably to hotel guests in ways that they could plausibly claim a moral authority. The floor staff in the nursing homes, rather than positioning themselves against the "customers" (i.e., residents), constructed a symbolic hierarchy of caring to claim a higher status than the managers.

NOTES TO CHAPTER 4

1. Kuttner, 1999; Mahar, 2006; Relman, 1980.

2. DiMaggio and Powell, 1983; Meyer and Rowan, 1977.

3. DiMaggio and Powell, 1983.

4. Levinson, 2010.

5. Residents are grouped into categories called resource utilization groups, or RUGs. The group each resident falls into is determined based on how much rehabilitation therapy the resident receives and how many activities of daily living he or she needs help with. The higher the classification, the more Medicare pays.

6. Levinson, 2010: ii.

7. Levinson, 2010: 11.

8. Medicare Payment Advisory Commission, 2011.

9. I do not know how much of those extra costs are offset by not having to provide benefits packages to the agency staff.

10. There is empirical evidence to support this claim (Kruzich, Clinton, et al., 1992; Pekkarinen, Sinervo, et al., 2004).

11. Castle, 2006.

12. The other units, by comparison, were more behaviorally oriented than clinically oriented.

13. Mahar, 2006.

14. DiMaggio and Powell, 1983.

NOTES TO CHAPTER 5

1. Abbasi and Rudman, 1994.

2. Suominen, Muurinen, et al., 2005.

3. Pirlich and Lochs, 2001.

4. Nijs, de Graaf, et al., 2006.

5. Mathey, Vanneste, et al., 2001.
6. Crogan and Pasvogel, 2003; Kane, 2001.
7. Evans, Crogan, et al., 2005.
8. DeVault, 1994.
9. Crogan, Evans, et al., 2004.
10. Kowanko, Simon, et al., 1999; Shultz, Crogan, et al., 2006.
11. Kayser-Jones, 1996: 27.
12. Sidenvall, 1999.
13. Bryon, de Casterle, et al., 2008.
14. At a 95 percent confidence interval.
15. Family members were sent surveys to respond on behalf of residents who were unable to respond.
16. Schwartz, 1978.
17. Since Marilyn could not give consent due to her dementia, Rolling Hills was authorized to do this. Otherwise, residents are allowed to refuse medications and make decisions that may harm their health.
18. Evans, Crogan, et al., 2005.
19. Pedersen, 2005.
20. Crogan, Evans, et al., 2004.
21. Mathey, Siebelink, et al., 2001.

NOTES TO CHAPTER 6

1. An earlier version of this chapter was published as an article in *Sociological Forum* (Rodriquez, 2011).
2. Hodson, 2001; Hodson and Roscigno, 2004; Lamont, 2000; Newman, 2000.
3. Glenn, 2000.
4. Hochschild, 1979, 1983.
5. Karakayali, 2009.
6. Swidler, 2003.
7. Lief and Fox, 1963; Smith and Kleinman, 1989.
8. Pulsford and Duxbury, 2006.
9. Geertz, 1973: 18.
10. Hochschild, 1983.
11. At various points in my fieldwork I asked staff members—floor staff and managers—if there was ever any training about how to show care for residents, for example, about whether to address them by their first name, their last name, or perhaps even their nickname, or whether anyone emphasized that residents should be dressed in clothes that match. I received a lot of blank stares as replies. Using forms of care that show emotional investment in the well-being of residents was not something that was trained so much as it was learned through working on the job.
12. Bone 2002:146
13. Lopez, 2006a.
14. Hochschild, 1979, 1983.
15. Smith-Lovin, 1998.

16. Leidner, 1993.
17. Wharton, 1993: 205.
18. Tolich, 1993.
19. Paules, 1991.
20. Hodson, 2001: 4.
21. Stacey, 2011.
22. Clark, 1987; Lawler and Yoon, 1996.

NOTES TO CHAPTER 7

1. An earlier version of this chapter was published as an article in *Social Psychology Quarterly* (Rodriquez, 2009).
2. Cohen-Mansfield and Lipson, 2008; Fagerlin and Schneider, 2004; McAuley and Travis, 2003; Resnick, Schuur, et al., 2009; Weinick, Wilcox, et al., 2008.
3. Gubrium, 1975.
4. Pollner and McDonald-Wikler, 1985.
5. Weinberg, 1997.
6. Gubrium, 1986; Mead, 1934.
7. Scott and Lyman, 1968.
8. Hochschild, 1983.
9. Akerstrom, 2002.
10. Emanuel, Ferris, et al., 2009: 12, emphasis in original.
11. Research about the extent to which individuals can time their death is limited and mixed. *Final Gifts* (Callanan and Kelley, 1992) explores dying from the perspective of hospice workers and works from an assumption that patients are "individuals with control over their living and dying" (23). On a larger scale, sociologists Phillips and Smith (1990) found morbidity among the Chinese to decrease by 35 percent the week prior to the Harvest Moon Festival and increase by the same amount the following week. However, these findings are countered by epidemiological studies, which have found no significant relationship between meaningful occasions and temporal variation in mortality. A recent analysis (Young and Hade, 2004) of 1.2 million death certificates from Ohio found that the proportion of persons dying the week before a significant occasion such as a birthday or holiday was no different from the proportion of those dying afterward. Furthermore, a review article (Skala and Freedland, 2004) found no direct evidence showing that dying individuals "hold on" or "give in" around symbolically important events.
12. Seale, 1998.
13. Goffman, 1961.
14. Snyder, Chen, et al., 2007.
15. McPhaul and Lipscomb, 2004.
16. Gates, Fitzwater, et al., 1999; Pulsford and Duxbury, 2006.
17. Sloane, Hoeffer, et al., 2004.
18. Bud's wife disagreed with this decision and maintained that he did not have dementia.
19. Scott and Lyman, 1968.
20. Irvine, 1999; Stearns and Stearns, 1986.

21. McAdams, 2006.

22. Gubrium, 1975.

23. Callanan and Kelley, 1992; Corless, 1994.

24. Saunders, 1967.

25. McKhann, Drachman, et al., 1984.

26. Hochschild, 1983.

27. Evers, Tomic, et al., 2001, 2002.

28. Strumpf and Tomes, 1993.

29. Weiner, Freiman, et al., 2007.

NOTES TO CHAPTER 8

1. Castle and Engberg, 2006; Harrington, Woolhandler, et al., 2001; Hillmer, Wodchis, et al., 2005; Mor, Zinn, et al., 2004; O'Neill, Harrington, et al., 2003; Schlesinger and Gray, 2006; Spector, Selden, et al., 1998.

2. Centers for Medicare & Medicaid Services, 2014.

3. Reeves and Ford, 2004: 300.

4. Relman, 1980.

5. Mahar, 2006.

6. Zimmerman, 2003.

7. Degenholtz, Kane, et al., 2006.

8. Rahman and Applebaum, 2009: 731.

9. Lopez, 2006a.

10. Medicare Payment Advisory Commission, 2011.

11. Mor, Zinn, et al., 2004.

12. Quality of life refers to a broader set of experiences outside of narrower concepts such as quality of care or clinical outcomes. These include a sense of security, physical comforts, meaningful relationships, dignity, autonomy, and spiritual well-being. Quality of life is an inherently subjective experience that is likely best evaluated by nursing home residents directly, but regulators collect the information that is available on quality of life from staff assessments instead. This generates standard procedures of care that deaden and limit the breadth of the human experience—ones that reduce life in nursing homes to a banal daily existence where quality is measured in narrowly quantified ways.

13. Kane, 2001, 2003.

14. http://www.pioneernetwork.net/CultureChange/Whatis/.

15. Miller, Miller, et al., 2010.

16. Loe and Moore, 2012; Rabig, Thomas, et al., 2006.

17. Lopez, 2006a.

18. Doty, Koren, et al., 2008.

19. Capitman, Leutz, et al., 2005: 33.

20. Rahman and Schnelle, 2008.

21. Miller, Miller, et al., 2010.

22. Miller, Miller, et al., 2010: 65S.

23. Barry, Brannon, et al., 2005.

24. Anderson, Issel, et al., 2003.

25. Bishop, Weinberg, et al., 2008.

26. Doty, Koren, et al., 2008.

27. Yeatts and Cready, 2007: 337.

28. Angelelli, 2006.

29. Doty, Koren, et al., 2008.

30. Tyler and Parker, 2011.

31. Lopez, 2006b.

32. Castle, 2006.

33. Swidler, 1986, 2003.

34. Hochschild, 1983.

35. England, 2005.

36. Hodson, 2001; Lamont, 2000; Sherman, 2005, 2007; Stacey, 2005.

37. Lamont, 2000: 3.

38. Sherman, 2005.

39. Mead, 1934.

NOTES TO THE APPENDIX

1. Fleming, Evans, et al., 2003.

2. Haber and Gratton, 1994.

3. Ogden and Adams, 2009.

4. Quadagno, 1988.

5. Fleming, Evans, et al., 2003.

6. Holstein and Cole, 1996.

7. Initially, only hospital construction was included in the legislation. Nursing homes, rehabilitation facilities, and outpatient hospital departments were included in 1954.

8. Institute of Medicine, Committee on Nursing Home Regulation, 1986: Appendix A.

9. Mendelson, 1974; Vladeck, 1980.

10. Institute of Medicine, Committee on Nursing Home Regulation, 1986.

11. Quoted in Institute of Medicine, Committee on Nursing Home Regulation, 1986: 240.

12. Ogden and Adams, 2009.

13. Ogden and Adams, 2009.

14. Haber and Gratton, 1994.

15. Walshe, 2001.

16. Vladeck, 1980.

17. Institute of Medicine, Committee on Nursing Home Regulation, 1986.

18. Hawes, 1997.

19. "Rights for the Aged, Long Overdue," 1988.

20. Weiner, Freiman, et al., 2007; Zhang and Grabowski, 2004.

21. Ogden and Adams, 2009.

22. General Accounting Office, 1998.

23. Institute of Medicine, Committee on Improving the Quality of Long-Term Care, 2001.

REFERENCES

Abbasi, Adil A. and Daniel Rudman. 1994. "Undernutrition in the Nursing Home: Prevalence, Consequences, Causes and Prevention." *Nutrition Reviews* 52:113–122.

Akerstrom, Malin. 2002. "Slaps, Punches, Pinches—but Not Violence: Boundary Work in Nursing Homes for the Elderly." *Symbolic Interaction* 25:515–536.

Amirkhanyan, Anna A., Hyun Joon Kim, and Kristina T. Lambright. 2008. "Does the Public Sector Outperform the Nonprofit and For-Profit Sectors? Evidence from a National Panel Study on Nursing Home Quality and Access." *Journal of Policy Analysis and Management* 27:326–353.

Anderson, Randy I., Danielle Lewis, and James R. Webb. 1999. "The Efficiency of Nursing Home Chains and the Implications of Non-profit Status." *Journal of Real Estate Portfolio Management* 5:235–245.

Anderson, Ruth A., Michele L. Issel, and Reuben R. McDaniel. 2003. "Nursing Homes as Complex Adaptive Systems: Relationship between Management Practice and Resident Outcomes." *Nursing Research* 52:12–21.

Angelelli, Joe. 2006. "Promising Models for Transforming Long-Term Care." *Gerontologist* 46:428–430.

Ashforth, Blake E. and Glen E. Kreiner. 1999. "'How Can You Do It?' Dirty Work and the Challenge of Constructing a Positive Identity." *Academy of Management Review* 24:413–434.

Barry, Theresa, Diane Brannon, and Vincent Mor. 2005. "Nurse Aide Empowerment Strategies and Staff Stability: Effects on Nursing Home Resident Outcomes." *Gerontologist* 45:309–317.

Bishop, Christine E., Marie R. Squillace, Jennifer Meagher, Wayne L. Anderson, and Joshua M. Wiener. 2009. "Nursing Home Work Practices and Nursing Assistants' Job Satisfaction." *Gerontologist* 49:611–622.

Bishop, Christine E., Dana Beth Weinberg, Walter Leutz, Almas Dossa, Susan G. Pfefferle, and Rebekah M. Zincavage. 2008. "Nursing Assistants' Job Commitment: Effect of Nursing Home Organizational Factors and Impact on Resident Well-Being." *Gerontologist* 48:36–45.

Black, Helen K. and Robert L. Rubinstein. 2005. "Direct Care Workers' Response to Dying and Death in the Nursing Home: A Case Study." *Journals of Gerontology Series B: Psychological Sciences and Social Sciences* 60:S3–S10.

Bone, Debora. 2002. "Dilemmas of Emotion Work in Nursing under Market-Driven Health Care." *International Journal of Public Sector Management* 15:140–150.

Bowers, Barbara J., Sarah Esmond, and Nora Jacobson. 2000. "The Relationship between Staffing and Quality in Long-Term Care Facilities: Exploring the Views of Nurse Aides." *Journal of Nursing Care Quality* 14:55–64.

Brauer, Carmen A., Marcelo Coca-Perraillon, David M. Cutler, and Allisson B. Rosen. 2009. "Incidence and Mortality of Hip Fractures in the United States." *Journal of the American Medical Association* 302:1573–1579.

Bryon, Els, Bernadette Dierckx de Casterle, Chris Gastmans, Els Steeman, and Koen Milisen. 2008. "Mealtime Care on a Geriatric-Psychiatric Ward from the Perspective of the Caregivers: A Qualitative Case Study Design." *Issues in Mental Health Nursing* 29:471–494.

Bureau of Labor Statistics. 2008–2009. *Occupational Outlook Handbook: Nursing, Psychiatric, and Home Health Aides.* Edited by the U.S. Department of Labor. Washington, DC: U.S. Department of Labor.

———. 2012a. "Occupational Employment and Wages: Nursing Assistants. U.S. Bureau of Labor Statistics." In *Occupational Employment Statistics. May 2012.* Washington, DC: U.S. Department of Labor.

———. 2012b. "Occupational Outlook Handbook: Nursing Aides, Orderlies, and Attendants. U.S. Bureau of Labor Statistics." In *Occupational Outlook Handbook, 2012–13 Edition.* Washington, DC: U.S. Department of Labor.

———. 2014a. "Licensed Practical and Licensed Vocational Nurses." In *Occupational Outlook Handbook, 2014–15 Edition.* Washington, DC: U.S. Department of Labor, Bureau of Labor Statistics. http://www.bls.gov/ooh/healthcare/licensed-practical-and-licensed-vocational-nurses.htm.

———. 2014b. "Registered Nurses." In *Occupational Outlook Handbook, 2014–15 Edition.* Washington, DC: U.S. Department of Labor, Bureau of Labor Statistics. http://www.bls.gov/ooh/healthcare/registered-nurses.htm.

Callanan, Maggie and Patricia Kelley. 1992. *Final Gifts: Understanding the Special Awareness, Needs, and Communication of the Dying.* New York: Bantam Books.

Cancian, Francesca M. 2000. "Paid Emotional Care." In *Care Work: Gender, Labor, and the Welfare State,* edited by M. Harrington Meyer. New York: Routledge.

Capitman, John, Walter Leutz, Christine Bishop, and Rosemary Casler. 2005. *Long-Term Care Quality: Historical Overview and Current Initiatives.* Washington, DC: National Commission for Quality Long-Term Care.

Castle, Nicholas G. 2006. "Measuring Staff Turnover in Nursing Homes." *Gerontologist* 46:210–219.

Castle, Nicholas G. and John Engberg. 2006. "Organizational Characteristics Associated with Staff Turnover in Nursing Homes." *Gerontologist* 46:62–73.

Centers for Medicare & Medicaid Services. 2014. "National Health Expenditures by Type of Service and Source of Funds, CY 1960–2012." http://www.cms.gov/Research-Statistics-Data-and-Systems/Statistics-Trends-and-Reports/NationalHealthExpendData/NationalHealthAccountsHistorical.html.

Clark, Candace. 1987. "Sympathy Biography and Sympathy Margin." *American Journal of Sociology* 93:290–321.

Cohen-Mansfield, Jiska and Steven Lipson. 2008. "Which Advance Directive Matters? An Analysis of End-of-Life Decisions Made in Nursing Homes." *Research on Aging* 30:74–92.

Collins, James W., Laurie Wolf, Jennifer Bell, and Bradley Evanoff. 2004. "An Evaluation of a 'Best Practices' Musculoskeletal Injury Prevention Program in Nursing Homes." *Injury Prevention* 10:206–211.

Corless, Inge. 1994. "Dying Well: Symptom Control within Hospice Care." *Annual Review of Nursing Research* 12:125–146.

Crogan, Neva L., Bronwynne Evans, Billie Severtsen, and Jill A. Shultz. 2004. "Improving Nursing Home Food Service: Uncovering the Meaning of Food through Residents' Stories." *Journal of Gerontological Nursing* 30:29–36.

Crogan, Neva L. and Alice Pasvogel. 2003. "The Influence of Protein-Calorie Malnutrition on Quality of Life in Nursing Homes." *Journals of Gerontology Series A: Biological Sciences and Medical Sciences* 58:M159–M164.

Degenholtz, Howard B., Rosalie A. Kane, Robert L. Kane, Boris Bershadsky, and Kristen C. Kling. 2006. "Predicting Nursing Facility Residents' Quality of Life Using External Indicators." *Health Services Research* 41:335–356.

Denzin, Norman. 1989. *The Research Act: A Theoretical Introduction to Research Methods.* Englewood Cliffs, NJ: Prentice Hall.

DeVault, Marjorie L. 1994. *Feeding the Family: The Social Organization of Caring as Gendered Work.* Chicago: University of Chicago Press.

Diamond, Timothy. 1992. *Making Gray Gold: Narratives of Nursing Home Care.* Chicago: University of Chicago Press.

Dill, Janette S., Jennifer Craft Morgan, and Thomas R. Konrad. 2010. "Strengthening the Long-Term Care Workforce." *Journal of Applied Gerontology* 29:196–214.

DiMaggio, Paul J. and Walter W. Powell. 1983. "The Iron Cage Revisited: Institutional Isomorphism and Collective Rationality in Organizational Fields." *American Sociological Review* 48:147–160.

Dodson, Lisa and Rebekah M. Zincavage. 2007. "'It's Like a Family': Caring Labor, Exploitation, and Race in Nursing Homes." *Gender & Society* 21:905–928.

Doty, Michelle M., Mary Jane Koren, and Elizabeth L. Sturla. 2008. "*Culture Change in Nursing Homes: How Far Have We Come? Findings from the Commonwealth Fund 2007 National Survey of Nursing Homes.*" New York: Commonwealth Fund.

Duncan, Marie T. and David L. Morgan. 1994. "Sharing the Caring: Family Caregivers' Views of Their Relationships with Nursing Home Staff." *Gerontologist* 34:235–244.

Emanuel, Linda L., Frank D. Ferris, Charles F. Von Gunten, and Jamie Von Roenn. 2009. "The Last Hours of Living: Practical Advice for Clinicians." *Journal of GMC–Nepal* 2:6–21. http://www.gmc.edu.np/journals/vol2_issue2/the_last_hours_of_living_practical_advice_for_clinicians.pdf.

England, Paula. 2005. "Emerging Theories of Care Work." *Annual Review of Sociology* 31:381–399.

England, Paula, Michelle Budig, and Nancy Folbre. 2002. "Wages of Virtue: The Relative Pay of Care Work." *Social Problems* 49:455–473.

Evans, Bronwynne C., Neva L. Crogan, and Jill A. Shultz. 2005. "Innovations in Long-Term Care. The Meaning of Mealtimes: Connection to the Social World of the Nursing Home." *Journal of Gerontological Nursing* 31:11–17.

Evans, Rhonda D. and Dianne A. Porche. 2005. "The Nature and Frequency of Medicare/ Medicaid Fraud and Neutralization Techniques among Speech, Occupational, and Physical Therapists." *Deviant Behavior* 26:253–270.

Evers, Will, Welko Tomic, and Andre Brouwers. 2001. "Effects of Aggressive Behavior and Perceived Self-Efficacy on Burnout among Staff of Homes for the Elderly." *Issues in Mental Health Nursing* 22:439–454.

———. 2002. "Aggressive Behaviour and Burnout among Staff of Homes for the Elderly." *International Journal of Mental Health Nursing* 11:2–9.

Fagerlin, Angela and Carl E. Schneider. 2004. "Enough: The Failure of the Living Will." *Hastings Center Report* 34:30–42.

Federal Interagency Forum on Aging Related Statistics. 2010. *Older Americans 2010: Key Indicators of Well-Being*. Washington, DC: Government Printing Office.

Fleming, Kevin C., Jonathan M. Evans, and Darryl S. Chutka. 2003. "A Cultural and Economic History of Old Age in America." *Mayo Clinic Proceedings* 78:914–921.

Folbre, Nancy. 2001. *The Invisible Heart: Economics and Family Values*. New York: New Press.

Foner, Nancy. 1994. *The Caregiving Dilemma: Work in an American Nursing Home*. Berkeley: University of California Press.

Gates, Donna M., Evelyn Fitzwater, and Ursula Meyer. 1999. "Violence against Caregivers in Nursing Homes. Expected, Tolerated, and Accepted." *Journal of Gerontological Nursing* 25:12–22.

Gates, Donna, Evelyn Fitzwater, Suzanne Telintelo, Paul Succop, and Marilyn S. Sommers. 2004. "Preventing Assaults by Nursing Home Residents: Nursing Assistants' Knowledge and Confidence—A Pilot Study." *Journal of the American Medical Directors Association* 5:S17–S21.

Geertz, Clifford. 1973. *The Interpretation of Cultures*. New York: Basic Books.

General Accounting Office. 1998. *California Nursing Homes: Care Problems Persist Despite Federal and State Oversight*. GAO/HEHS-98-202. Washington, DC: General Accounting Office.

Genworth. 2013. *Executive Summary: Genworth 2013: Cost of Care Survey: Home Care Providers, Adult Day Health Care Facilities, Assisted Living Facilities and Nursing Homes*. 10th ed. Richmond, VA: Genworth Financial.

Gessert, Charles E., Irina V. Haller, Robert L. Kane, and Howard Degenholtz. 2006. "Rural–Urban Differences in Medical Care for Nursing Home Residents with Severe Dementia at the End of Life." *Journal of the American Geriatrics Society* 54:1199–1205.

Gittler, Josephine. 2008. "Governmental Efforts to Improve Quality of Care for Nursing Home Residents and to Protect Them from Mistreatment: A Survey of Federal and State Laws." *Research in Gerontological Nursing* 1:264–284.

Glenn, Evelyn Nakano. 2000. "Creating a Caring Society." *Contemporary Sociology* 29:84–94.

Goffman, Erving. 1959. *The Presentation of Self in Everyday Life*. New York: Doubleday.

———. 1961. *Asylums: Essays on the Social Situation of Mental Patients and Other Inmates.* New York: Doubleday.

Gubrium, Jaber. 1975. *Living and Dying at Murray Manor.* New York: St. Martin's.

———. 1986. "The Social Preservation of Mind: The Alzheimer's Disease Experience." *Symbolic Interaction* 9:37–51.

Haber, Carole and Brian Gratton. 1994. *Old Age and the Search for Security: An American Social History.* Bloomington: Indiana University Press.

Hannan, Shirina, Ian J. Norman, and Sally J. Redfern. 2001. "Care Work and Quality of Care for Older People: A Review of the Research Literature." *Reviews in Clinical Gerontology* 11:189–203.

Harrington, Charlene, Helen Carrillo, and Brandee Woleslagle Blank. 2008. *Nursing Home Facilities, Staffing, Residents, and Facility Deficiencies, 2001 through 2007.* San Francisco: Department of Social and Behavioral Sciences, University of California, San Francisco.

Harrington, Charlene, Steffie Woolhandler, Joseph Mullan, Helen Carrillo, and David U. Himmelstein. 2001. "Does Investor Ownership of Nursing Homes Compromise the Quality of Care?" *American Journal of Public Health* 91:1452–1455.

Harrington Meyer, Madonna, ed. 2000. *Care Work: Gender, Class, and the Welfare State.* New York: Routledge.

Hawes, Catherine. 1997. "Regulation and the Politics of Long-Term Care." *Generations* 21:5–9.

He, Wan, Manisha Sengupta, Victoria A. Velkoff, and Kimberly A. Debarros. 2005. "65+ in the United States." In *Current Population Reports*, edited by the U.S. Census Bureau. Washington, DC: U.S. Census Bureau.

Hillmer, Michael P., Walter P. Wodchis, Sudeep Gill, Geoffrey Anderson, and Paula A. Rochon. 2005. "Nursing Home Profit Status and Quality of Care: Is There Any Evidence of an Association?" *Medical Care Research and Review* 62:139–166.

Himmelweit, Susan. 1999. "Caring Labor." *Annals of the American Academy of Political and Social Science* 56:27–38.

Hochschild, Arlie Russell. 1979. "Emotion Work, Feeling Rules, and Social Structure." *American Journal of Sociology* 85:551–575.

———. 1983. *The Managed Heart: Commercialization of Human Feeling.* Berkeley: University of California Press.

———. 2013. *The Outsourced Self: What Happens When We Pay Others to Live Our Lives for Us.* New York: Picador Press.

Hodson, Randy. 2001. *Dignity at Work.* Cambridge: Cambridge University Press.

Hodson, Randy and Vincent J. Roscigno. 2004. "Organizational Success and Worker Dignity: Complementary or Contradictory?" *American Journal of Sociology* 110:672–708.

Holstein, Martha and Thomas R. Cole. 1996. "The Evolution of Long-Term Care in America." In *The Future of Long-Term Care: Social and Policy Issues*, edited by Robert H. Binstock, Leighton C. Cluff, and Otto von Mering. Baltimore: Johns Hopkins University Press.

Horn, Susan D., Peter Buerhaus, Nancy Bergstrom, and Randall J. Smout. 2005. "RN Staffing Time and Outcomes of Long-Stay Nursing Home Residents: Pressure Ulcers and Other

Adverse Outcomes Are Less Likely as RNs Spend More Time on Direct Patient Care." *American Journal of Nursing* 105:58–70.

Hughes, Everett C. 1951. "Work and the Self." In *Social Psychology at the Crossroads*, edited by J. H. Rohrer and M. Sherif. New York: Harper.

———. 1958. *Men and Their Work*. Glencoe, IL: Free Press.

Institute of Medicine, Committee on Improving the Quality of Long-Term Care. 2001. *Improving the Quality of Long-term Care*. Washington, DC: National Academies Press.

Institute of Medicine, Committee on Nursing Home Regulation. 1986. *Improving the Quality of Care in Nursing Homes*. Washington, DC: National Academies Press.

Irvine, Leslie. 1999. *Codependent Forevermore: The Invention of Self in a Twelve Step Group*. Chicago: University of Chicago Press.

Jones, Adrienne L., Lisa L. Dwyer, Anita R. Bercovitz, and Genevieve W. Strahan. 2009. "The National Nursing Home Survey: 2004 Overview." *Vital and Health Statistics. Series 13, Data from the National Health Survey* 13(167):1–155.

Kaffenberger, K. R. 2001. "Nursing Home Ownership—An Historical Analysis." *Journal of Aging & Social Policy* 12:35–48.

Kaiser Commission on Medicaid and the Uninsured. 2013. "Overview of Nursing Facility Capacity, Financing, and Ownership in the United States in 2011." Kaiser Family Foundation. http://kaiserfamilyfoundation.files.wordpress.com/2013/06/8456-overview-of-nursing-facility-capacity.pdf.

Kane, Rosalie A. 2001. "Long-Term Care and a Good Quality of Life." *Gerontologist* 41:293–304.

———. 2003. "Definition, Measurement, and Correlates of Quality of Life in Nursing Homes: Toward a Reasonable Practice, Research, and Policy Agenda." *Gerontologist* 43:28–36.

Karakayali, Nedim. 2009. "Social Distance and Affective Orientations." *Sociological Forum* 24:538–562.

Kassirer, Jerome P. 2005. *On The Take: How Medicine's Complicity with Big Business Can Endanger Your Health*. New York: Oxford University Press.

Kayser-Jones, Jeanie. 1996. "Mealtime in Nursing Homes: The Importance of Individualized Care." *Journal of Gerontological Nursing* 22:26–31.

Kemp, Candace L., Mary M. Ball, Molly M. Perkins, Carole Hollingsworth, and Michael J. Lepore. 2009. "'I Get Along with Most of Them': Direct Care Workers' Relationships with Residents' Families in Assisted Living." *Gerontologist* 49:224–235.

Knox, Kris J., Eric C. Blankmeyer, and J. R. Stutzman. 2001. "The Efficiency of Nursing Home Chains and the Implications of Nonprofit Status: A Comment." *Journal of Real Estate Portfolio Management* 7:177–182.

Kowanko, Inge, Stephen Simon, and Jacquelin Wood. 1999. "Nutritional Care of the Patient: Nurses' Knowledge and Attitudes in an Acute Care Setting." *Journal of Clinical Nursing* 8:217–224.

Kruzich, Jean M., Jacqueline F. Clinton, and Sheryl T. Kelber. 1992. "Personal and Environmental Influences on Nursing Home Satisfaction." *Gerontologist* 32:342–350.

Kuttner, Robert. 1999. *Everything for Sale: The Virtues and Limits of Markets.* Chicago: University of Chicago Press.

Lamont, Michele. 2000. *The Dignity of Working Men: Morality and the Boundaries of Race, Class, and Immigration.* New York: Russell Sage Foundation.

Lamont, Michele and Virag Molnar. 2002. "The Study of Boundaries in the Social Sciences." *Annual Review of Sociology* 28:167–195.

Lawler, Edward J. and Jeongkoo Yoon. 1996. "Commitment in Exchange Relations: Test of a Theory of Relational Cohesion." *American Sociological Review* 61:89–108.

Lee Treweek, Geraldine. 1996. "Emotion Work, Order and Emotional Power in Care Assistant Work." In *Health and the Sociology of Emotions*, edited by Veronica James and Jonathon Gabe. Oxford: Blackwell.

Leidner, Robin. 1993. *Fast Food, Fast Talk: Service Work and the Routinization of Everyday Life.* Berkeley: University of California Press.

Levinson, Daniel R. 2008. "Trends in Nursing Home Deficiencies and Complaints" (OEI-02-08-00 140). Washington, DC: Office of Inspector General, Department of Health and Human Services.

———. 2010. *Questionable Billing by Skilled Nursing Facilities* (OEI-02-09-00202). Washington, DC: Office of Inspector General, Department of Health and Human Services.

Lief, Harold I. and Renee C. Fox. 1963. "Training for 'Detached Concern' in Medical Students." In *The Psychological Basis of Medical Practice*, edited by Harold I. Lief. New York: Harper and Row.

Lipsky, Michael. 2010. *Street-Level Bureaucracy: Dilemmas of the Individual in Public Services.* New York: Russell Sage Foundation.

Loe, Meika and Crystal Dea Moore. 2012. "From Nursing Home to Green House: Changing Contexts of Eldercare in the United States." *Journal of Applied Gerontology* 31:755–763.

Lopez, Steven H. 2006a. "Culture Change Management in Long-Term Care: A Shop Floor View." *Politics and Society* 34:55–79.

———. 2006b. "Emotional Labor and Organized Emotional Care: Conceptualizing Nursing Home Care Work." *Work and Occupations* 33:133–160.

Mahar, Maggie. 2006. *Money-Driven Medicine: The Real Reason Health Care Costs So Much.* New York: HarperCollins.

Martin, Kitchener, Janis O'Meara, Brody Ab, Lee Hyang Yuol, and Charlene Harrington. 2008. "Shareholder Value and the Performance of a Large Nursing Home Chain." *Health Services Research* 43:1062–1084.

Mathey, Marie-Françoise A. M., Els Siebelink, Cees de Graaf, and Wya A. Van Staveren. 2001. "Flavor Enhancement of Food Improves Dietary Intake and Nutritional Status of Elderly Nursing Home Residents." *Journals of Gerontology Series A: Biological Sciences* 56:M200–M205.

Mathey, Marie-Françoise A. M., Vincent G. G. Vanneste, Cees de Graaf, Lisette C. P. G. M. De Groot, and Wija A. Van Staveren. 2001. "Health Effect of Improved Meal Ambiance in a Dutch Nursing Home: A 1-Year Intervention Study." *Preventive Medicine* 32:416–423.

McAdams, Dan P. 2006. *The Redemptive Self: Stories Americans Live By*. Oxford: Oxford University Press.

McAuley, William J. and Shirley S. Travis. 2003. "Advance Care Planning among Residents in Long-Term Care." *American Journal of Hospice and Palliative Medicine* 20:353–359.

McKhann, Guy, David Drachman, Marshall Folstein, Robert Katzman, Donald Price, and Emanuel M. Stadlan. 1984. "Clinical Diagnosis of Alzheimer's Disease: Report of the NINCDS-ADRDA Work Group, under the Auspices of Department of Health and Human Services Task Force on Alzheimer's Disease." *Neurology* 34:939–943.

McPhaul, Kathleen M. and Jane A. Lipscomb. 2004. "Workplace Violence in Health Care: Recognized but Not Regulated." *Online Journal of Issues in Nursing* 9(3):6. http://www.nursingworld.org/MainMenuCategories/ANAMarketplace/ANAPeriodicals/OJIN/TableofContents/Volume92004/No3Sept04/ViolenceinHealthcare.html.

Mead, George Herbert. 1934. *Mind, Self and Society: From the Standpoint of a Social Behaviorist*. Chicago: University of Chicago Press.

Medicare Payment Advisory Commission. 2011. "Report to the Congress." Edited by Medicare Payment Advisory Commission. Washington, DC: Medicare Payment Advisory Commission.

Mendelson, Mary Adelaide. 1974. *Tender Loving Greed: How the Incredibly Lucrative Nursing Home "Industry" Is Exploiting America's Old People and Defrauding Us All*. New York: Knopf.

Meyer, John W. and Brian Rowan. 1977. "Institutionalized Organizations: Formal Structure as Myth and Ceremony." *American Journal of Sociology* 83:340–363.

Miller, Edward A. and Vincent Mor. 2006. "Out of the Shadows: Envisioning a Brighter Future for Long-Term Care in America." Brown University Report for the National Commission for Quality Long Term Care. Providence, RI: Brown University.

Miller, Susan C., Edward Alan Miller, Hye-Young Jung, Samantha Sterns, Melissa Clark, and Vincent Mor. 2010. "Nursing Home Organizational Change: The 'Culture Change' Movement as Viewed by Long-Term Care Specialists." *Medical Care Research and Review* 67:65S–81S.

Mills, C. Wright. 1940. "Situated Actions and Vocabularies of Motive." *American Sociological Review* 5:904–913.

Mor, Vincent, Jacqueline Zinn, Joseph Angelelli, Joan M. Teno, and Susan C. Miller. 2004. "Driven to Tiers: Socioeconomic and Racial Disparities in the Quality of Nursing Home Care." *Milbank Quarterly* 82:227–256.

Moss, Miriam S., Sidney Z. Moss, Robert L. Rubinstein, and Helen K. Black. 2003. "The Metaphor of 'Family' in Staff Communication about Dying and Death." *Journals of Gerontology Series B: Psychological Sciences and Social Sciences* 58:S290–S296.

Newman, Katherine S. 2000. *No Shame in My Game: Working Poor in the Inner City*. New York: Vintage.

Nijs, Kristel, Cees de Graaf, Frans J. Kok, and Wija A. Van Staveren. 2006. "Effect of Family Style Mealtimes on Quality of Life, Physical Performance, and Body Weight of Nursing Home Residents: Cluster Randomised Controlled Trial." *British Medical Journal* 332:1180–1184.

Ogden, Lydia L. and Kathleen Adams. 2009. "Poorhouse to Warehouse: Institutional Long-Term Care in the United States." *Publius* 39:138–163.

O'Neill, Ciaran, Charlene Harrington, Martin Kitchener, and Debra Saliba. 2003. "Quality of Care in Nursing Homes: An Analysis of Relationships among Profit, Quality, and Ownership." *Medical Care* 41:1318–1330.

Paules, Greta Foff. 1991. *Dishing It Out: Power and Resistance among Waitresses in a New Jersey Restaurant*. Philadelphia: Temple University Press.

Pedersen, Preben Ulrich. 2005. "Nutritional Care: The Effectiveness of Actively Involving Older Patients." *Journal of Clinical Nursing* 14:247–255.

Pekkarinen, Laura, Timo Sinervo, Marja-Leena Perälä, and Marko Elovainio. 2004. "Work Stressors and the Quality of Life in Long-Term Care Units." *Gerontologist* 44:633–643.

Pennington, Karen, Jill Scott, and Kathy Magilvy. 2003. "The Role of Certified Nursing Assistants in Nursing Homes." *Journal of Nursing Administration* 33:578–584.

Penrod, Joan D. 2001. "Functional Disability at Nursing Home Admission: A Comparison of Urban and Rural Admission Cohorts." *Journal of Rural Health* 17:229–238.

Phillips, David and David Smith. 1990. "Postponement of Death until Symbolically Meaningful Occasions." *Journal of the American Medical Association* 63:1947–1951.

Pirlich, Matthias and Herbert Lochs. 2001. "Nutrition in the Elderly." *Best Practice & Research Clinical Gastroenterology* 15:869–884.

Pollner, Melvin and Lynn McDonald-Wikler. 1985. "The Social Construction of Unreality: A Case Study of a Family's Attribution of Competence to a Severely Retarded Child." *Family Process* 24:241–254.

Pulsford, Dave and Joy Duxbury. 2006. "Aggressive Behaviour by People with Dementia in Residential Care Settings: A Review." *Journal of Psychiatric and Mental Health Nursing* 13:611–618.

Quadagno, Jill. 1988. *The Transformation of Old Age Security: Class and Politics in the American Welfare State*. Chicago: University of Chicago Press.

Rabig, Judith, William Thomas, Rosalie A. Kane, Lois J. Cutler, and Steve McAlilly. 2006. "Radical Redesign of Nursing Homes: Applying the Green House Concept in Tupelo, Mississippi." *Gerontologist* 46:533–539.

Rahman, Anna N. and Robert A. Applebaum. 2009. "The Nursing Home Minimum Data Set Assessment Instrument: Manifest Functions and Unintended Consequences—Past, Present, and Future." *Gerontologist* 49:727–735.

Rahman, Anna N. and John F. Schnelle. 2008. "The Nursing Home Culture-Change Movement: Recent Past, Present, and Future Directions for Research." *Gerontologist* 48:142–148.

Reeves, Terry C. and Eric W. Ford. 2004. "Strategic Management and Performance Differences: Nonprofit versus For-Profit Health Organizations." *Health Care Management Review* 29:298–308.

Relman, Arnold S. 1980. "The New Medical-Industrial Complex." *New England Journal of Medicine* 303:963–970.

Resnick, Helaine E., Jeremiah D. Schuur, Janice Heineman, Robyn Stone, and Joel S. Weissman. 2009. "Advance Directives in Nursing Home Residents Aged > or =65 Years: United States 2004." *American Journal of Hospice and Palliative Medicine* 25:476–482.

"Rights for the Aged, Long Overdue." 1988. *New York Times*, January 19: A26.

Rodriquez, Jason. 2009. "Attributions of Agency and the Construction of Moral Order: Dementia, Death, and Dignity in Nursing-Home Care." *Social Psychology Quarterly* 72:165–179.

———. 2011. "'It's a Dignity Thing': Nursing Home Care Workers' Use of Emotions." *Sociological Forum* 26:265–286.

Saunders, Cecily. 1967. *The Management of Terminal Illness*. London: Hospital Medical.

Schein, Edgar H. 1990. "Organizational Culture." *American Psychologist* 45:109–119.

Schlesinger, Mark and Bradford H. Gray. 2006. "How Nonprofits Matter in American Medicine, and What to Do about It." *Health Affairs* 25:W287–W303.

Schwartz, Barry. 1978. "The Social Ecology of Time Barriers." *Social Forces* 56:1203–1220.

Scott, Marvin B. and Stanford M. Lyman. 1968. "Accounts." *American Sociological Review* 33:46–62.

Scott-Cawiezell, Jill, Katherine Jones, Laurie Moore, and Carol Vojir. 2005. "Nursing Home Culture: A Critical Component in Sustained Improvement." *Journal of Nursing Care Quality* 20:341–348.

Seale, Clive. 1998. *Constructing Death: The Sociology of Dying and Bereavement*. Cambridge: Cambridge University Press.

Sennett, Richard. 2009. *The Craftsman*. New Haven, CT: Yale University Press.

Sherman, Rachel. 2005. "Producing the Superior Self: Strategic Comparison and Symbolic Boundaries among Luxury Hotel Workers." *Ethnography* 6:131–158.

———. 2007. *Class Acts: Service and Inequality in Luxury Hotels*. Berkeley: University of California Press.

Shultz, Jill Armstrong, Neva L. Crogan, and Bronwynne C. Evans. 2006. "Organizational Issues Related to Satisfaction with Food and Food Service in the Nursing Home from the Resident's Perspective." *Journal of Nutrition in Gerontology and Geriatrics* 24:39–55.

Sidenvall, B. 1999. "Meal Procedures in Institutions for Elderly People: A Theoretical Interpretation." *Journal of Advanced Nursing* 30:319–328.

Skala, Judith and Kenneth Freedland. 2004. "Death Takes a Raincheck." *Psychosomatic Medicine* 66:382–386.

Sloane, Philip D., Beverly Hoeffer, C. Madeline Mitchell, Darlene A. McKenzie, Ann Louise Barrick, Joanne Rader, Barbara J. Stewart, Karen Amann Talerico, Joyce H. Rasin, Richard C. Zink, and Gary G. Koch. 2004. "Effect of Person-Centered Showering and the Towel Bath on Bathing-Associated Aggression, Agitation, and Discomfort in Nursing Home Residents with Dementia: A Randomized, Controlled Trial." *Journal of the American Geriatrics Society* 52:1795–1804.

Smith, Allen C. and Sherryl Kleinman. 1989. "Managing Emotions in Medical School: Students' Contacts with the Living and the Dead." *Social Psychology Quarterly* 52:56–69.

Smith-Lovin, Lynn. 1998. "Emotion Management as Emotional Labor." In *Required Reading: Sociology's Most Influential Books*, edited by D. Clawson. Amherst: University of Massachusetts Press.

Snyder, Lori Anderson, Peter Y. Chen, and Tammi Vacha-Haase. 2007. "The Underreporting Gap in Aggressive Incidents from Geriatric Patients against Certified Nursing Assistants." *Violence and Victims* 22:367–379.

Spector, William D., Thomas M. Selden, and Joel W. Cohen. 1998. "The Impact of Ownership Type on Nursing Home Outcomes." *Health Economics* 7:639–653.

Stacey, Clare L. 2005. "Finding Dignity in Dirty Work: The Constraints and Rewards of Low-Wage Home Care Labour." *Sociology of Health & Illness* 27:831–854.

———. 2011. *The Caring Self: The Work Experiences of Home Care Aides.* Ithaca, NY: Cornell University Press.

Starr, Paul. 1982. *The Social Transformation of American Medicine.* New York: Basic Books.

Stearns, Carol Zisowitz and Peter Stearns. 1986. *Anger: The Struggle for Emotional Control in America's History.* Chicago: University of Chicago Press.

Stevenson, David G. and David C. Grabowski. 2008. "Private Equity Investment and Nursing Home Care: Is It a Big Deal?" *Health Affairs* 27:1399–1408.

Stone, Deborah. 2000. "Caring by the Book." In *Care Work: Gender, Class, and the Welfare State,* edited by Madonna Harrington Meyer. New York: Routledge.

Stone, Robyn and Mary F. Harahan. 2010. "Improving the Long-Term Care Workforce Serving Older Adults." *Health Affairs* 29:109–115.

Strumpf, Neville and Nancy Tomes. 1993. "Restraining the Troublesome Patient: A Historical Perspective on a Contemporary Debate." *Nursing History Review* 1:3–24.

Suominen, Merja, Seija Muurinen, Pirkko Routasalo, Helena Soini, Irmeli Suur-Uski, Arja Peiponen, Harriet Finne-Soveri, and K. H. Pitkala. 2005. "Malnutrition and Associated Factors among Aged Residents in All Nursing Homes in Helsinki." *European Journal of Clinical Nutrition* 59:578–583.

Swan, James H., Charlene Harrington, Wendy Clemena, Ruth B. Pickard, Liatris Studer, and Susan K. Dewit. 2000. "Medicaid Nursing Facility Reimbursement Methods: 1979–1997." *Med Care Research Review* 57:361–378.

Swidler, Ann. 1986. "Culture in Action: Symbols and Strategies." *American Sociological Review* 51:273–286.

———. 2003. *Talk of Love: How Culture Matters.* Chicago: University of Chicago Press.

Sykes, Gresham M. and David Matza. 1957. "Techniques of Neutralization: A Theory of Delinquency." *American Sociological Review* 22:664–670.

Tolich, Martin B. 1993. "Alienating and Liberating Emotions at Work: Supermarket Clerks' Performance of Customer Service." *Journal of Contemporary Ethnography* 22:361–381.

Trice, Harrison M. 1993. *Occupational Subcultures in the Workplace.* Ithaca, NY: ILR Press.

Tyler, Denise A. and Victoria A. Parker. 2011. "Nursing Home Culture, Teamwork, and Culture Change." *Journal of Research in Nursing* 16:37–49.

Verbeek, Hilde, Sandra Zwakhalen, Erik Van Rossum, Ton Ambergen, Gertrudis Kempen, and Jan Hamers. 2010. "Small-Scale, Homelike Facilities versus Regular Psychogeriatric Nursing Home Wards: A Cross-Sectional Study into Residents' Characteristics." *BMC Health Services Research* 10(1):30–36.

Vladeck, Bruce. 1980. *Unloving Care: The Nursing Home Tragedy.* New York: Basic Books.

Walker, Nancy A. 1998. *What's So Funny? Humor in American Culture.* Wilmington, DE: Scholarly Resources.

Walshe, Kieran. 2001. "Regulating U.S. Nursing Homes: Are We Learning from Experience?" *Health Affairs* 20:128–144.

Weinberg, Darin. 1997. "The Social Construction of Non-human Agency: The Case of Mental Disorder." *Social Problems* 44:217–234.

Weiner, Joshua M., Marc P. Freiman, and David Brown. 2007. *Nursing Home Quality: Twenty Years after the Omnibus Budget Reconciliation Act of 1987.* Menlo Park, CA: Kaiser Family Foundation.

Weinick, Robin M., Susan R. Wilcox, Elyse R. Park, Richard T. Griffey, and Joel S. Weissman. 2008. "Use of Advance Directives for Nursing Home Residents in the Emergency Department." *American Journal of Hospice and Palliative Medicine* 25:179–183.

Wharton, Amy S. 1993. "The Affective Consequences of Service Work: Managing Emotions on the Job." *Work and Occupations* 20:205–232.

Williams, Christine L. 1992. "The Glass Escalator: Hidden Advantages for Men in the 'Female Professions.'" *Social Problems* 39:15.

Yeatts, Dale E. and Cynthia M. Cready. 2007. "Consequences of Empowered CNA Teams in Nursing Home Settings: A Longitudinal Assessment." *Gerontologist* 47:323–339.

Young, Donn and Erin Hade. 2004. "Holidays, Birthdays and Postponement of Cancer Death." *Journal of the American Medical Association* 292:3012–3016.

Zhang, Xinzhi and David C. Grabowski. 2004. "Nursing Home Staffing and Quality under the Nursing Home Reform Act." *Gerontologist* 44:13–23.

Zimmerman, David R. 2003. "Improving Nursing Home Quality of Care through Outcomes Data: The MDS Quality Indicators." *International Journal of Geriatric Psychiatry* 18:250–257.

ABOUT THE AUTHOR

Jason Rodriquez is Assistant Professor of Sociology at the University of Missouri–Columbia. He received his Ph.D. from the University of Massachusetts–Amherst and was an NIMH Post-Doctoral Fellow at the Rutgers University Institute for Health, Health Care Policy, and Aging Research. He is originally from Staten Island, New York.

Lightning Source UK Ltd.
Milton Keynes UK
UKOW02f0622210815

257301UK00003B/39/P